HELPING HUMANS ONE ANIMAL AT A TIME

STORIES & STUDIES OF ANIMALS, PLANTS & HUMAN COMPANIONS IMPROVING EACH OTHERS LIVES

MEG HARRISON

BALBOA.
PRESS

A DIVISION OF HAY HOUSE

Cover Art: Brett Stokes of Fallbrook, CA
Photo credit on page 152: Jaime Windon/Momenta Workshops

Balboa Press books may be ordered through booksellers or by contacting:

Balboa Press
A Division of Hay House
1663 Liberty Drive
Bloomington, IN 47403
www.balboapress.com
1-(877) 407-4847

Printed in the United States of America.

ISBN: 978-1-4525-7215-4 (sc)
ISBN: 978-1-4525-7252-9 (e)

Balboa Press rev. date: 04/26/2013

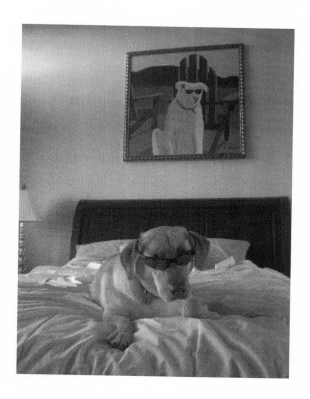

Here is my editor, Stella. She quit. She moved to Hollywood to write for Ellen. One quick postcard later, Stella said Ellen was much more fun and wished me 'good luck.'

I, the author, make no apologies for breaking the rules of grammar—which may have been the cause of Editor Stella running away—that and an open back gate. Nevertheless, moving on, I think Cat, Dog, Horse, and Flowers should all be capitalized whilst Stella strongly disagreed about capitalizing Cats.

And left on my own, I make up words, capitalize out of respect, and begin sentences with "And." Some of what you will read was previously published and fabulously edited by professionals. As for the rest, all I can say is if you are an English teacher; you are gonna run out of red ink. The rest of you, enjoy the diversity.

Table of Contents

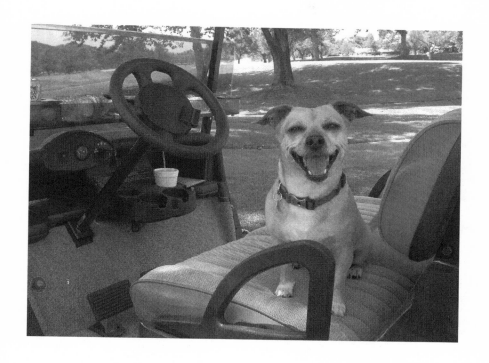

"Climb in. I'll drive. It'll be fun. Honest."

Why Are We Here?

Why are you reading this? Because you want to help. Pure and Simple—that's the answer. I wrote this for you. Because, for a long time, I had no one to share these amazing stories with—no one that would understand the depths of my sorrow when I could not help or the mystical feeling when I could. I want to share my stories with someone who wants to listen, to possibly take some of this hard-won experience and help others.

My experience has come at a cost, a pretty hefty price tag—both emotionally and financially. But, you will see through the stories and the studies—worth every teardrop and every dime.

There is a theory, a phenomena called: *The Hundredth Monkey*—also the title of a book written by Ken Keyes in 1982 concerning *Macaca fuscata* Monkeys living on the island of Koshima. In 1952, Japanese scientists observing these Monkeys started to feed them sweet potatoes dropped in the sand. The Monkeys liked the taste but not the dirt. One young female named Imo washed her potato in a stream. Then taught her mother. In the next 6 years, all the young ones washed their potatoes.

From *The Hundredth Monkey*: "Only the adults who imitated their children learned this SOCIAL IMPROVEMENT. Other adults kept eating dirty potatoes. Then something startling took place. In the autumn of 1958, a certain number of Koshima Monkeys were washing sweet potatoes—the exact number is not known. Let us suppose that when the sun rose one morning there were 99 Monkeys on Koshima Island who had learned to wash their sweet potatoes. Let's further suppose that later that morning, the 100th Monkey learned to wash potatoes.

Then it happened.

By that evening almost everyone in the tribe was washing sweet potatoes before eating them. The ADDED ENERGY of this 100th Monkey somehow created an IDEOLOGICAL BREAKTHROUGH!

But… the most surprising thing observed by these scientists was that the habit of washing sweet potatoes then SPONTANEOUSLY JUMPED over the sea. Colonies of Monkeys on other islands and the mainland troop of Monkeys at Takasakiyama (Japan) began washing their sweet potatoes!" The book, *Lifetide* by Lyall Watson, Bantam Books, 1980, provides more details.

What I walk away with is, if the SOCIAL IMPROVEMENT is good for the individual and then for the society; this IMPROVEMENT will create an IDEOLOGICAL BREAKTHROUGH and when a "critical number" is reached; the new behavior will SPONTANEOUSLY JUMP to the next population.

Before you throw this baby out with the bath water, consider MADD, Mothers Against Drunk Drivers, and her humble beginnings of one person carrying a message about driving drunk which has had a massive positive impact. Or Susan G. Komen's sister missing her sibling, a victim of breast cancer, started with an idea and now, "Race for the Cure" has raised an incredible amount of money and awareness. Thousands of similar examples exist where one person had one reason to talk to one person.

Someone had to start the dialogue or take the action to improve the lives of the tribe. (Whether they thought they needed the improvement or not.) Wash the first potato, hand out informational flyers, talk to neighbors, try something new to see if it actually works better than the old status quo. Something. That's why we're here: to learn more about Flowers, Weeds, and Trees improving lives.

**"Never doubt that a small group
of thoughtful, committed citizens
can change the world.
Indeed, it is the only thing
that ever has."**
Margaret Mead, social anthropologist.

100 Monkeys and Counting.

You came here to find
what you already have

and

You came here to learn
what you already know.

For All Intents and Purposes

Flower Essences Right Wrongs.

This simple statement says it all: Flower Essences right wrongs. I have dabbled in natural solutions for 40 years and settled on Flower Essences for one reason: they work. They work for humans, for animals, alcoholic teenagers, victims of violence, their perpetrators, as well as family members, and witnesses to these transgressions.

Essences work 100% of the time, are accessible, and cause no harm. So what's not to love? Well, there are those who could be jealous of such a simple solution to difficult and costly problems. And there are those who feel threatened by the thought of having to change their minds and accept a new idea.

Effective, permanent improvement with POSITIVE side effects.

Answers to problems faced by domesticated animals no matter what the behavior, situation, or circumstance is what I am after and what I have gotten from using Flower Essences. If we can't let the animals run free in the woods and grasslands allowing access to their emotional nutrition; then, you can bring it to them in the simplest form possible: Essences.

Here is a good place to remind ourselves why we use flower essences: to improve and prevent problematic behavior, attitudes, emotions, and patterns of learning **because they go to the root cause of mental and emotional problems, not suppressing or masking the problematic behaviors to resurface later.**

There is no substitute for patience, positive training, and understanding but sometimes we simply need to pull the lamp closer to get a better look at the cause of the discontent. Essences will allow you to illuminate, see from a different angle, presenting the opportunity to reflect on the animals' specific needs and effect a permanent change. Whether dealing with an excessive personality trait, an ingrained fear or a brand new experience, remedies can give us that moment of opportunity to make IT work—whatever your IT is at the time.

30 Minutes to Save A Life
Why?
Because we can.
How?
Flowers, Water, and Sunshine.

Regrettably, the #1 reason for euthanasia is behavior. A Border Collie living in an apartment. Buying the difficult dog a companion. Crating for 10 hours a day and again at night. Feeding crummy food that leaves them perpetually unsatisfied creating stress. Do the best you can and when in doubt get good advice. Advice that FEELS right for you, your family, and all you share your life with.

Crazy Dogs, feral Cats, and aggressive Elephants can all be treated successfully and permanently. These misunderstood animals are acting out possible emotional or mental pain but, often causing injury to themselves or others in the process. Essences will help. Two problems are #1 asking the person observing to accept the fact an innocuous flower actually helped. #2 problem is there is less money to be made preventing something rather than treating the symptoms of the problem. Don't shoot the messenger—look into the industries for yourself. In the meantime, use Essences on the worst cases and observe for 30 minutes. Guarantee the behavior will improve 99% of the time. Even if the damage is grossly pathological, seemingly hopeless conditions can be remedied more often than not. Worth a try.

Frequently Asked Questions

Keeping the message simple (and free from politics), these FAQs refer to Remedies primarily prepared according to the 80 year old traditions of Dr. Edward Bach. Ineffective "remedies" and counterfeits do exist.

What do Flower Essences do?
Permanently transform and improve problematic behavior, attitudes, emotions, patterns of learning allowing any animal to excel to their fullest potential. Chronic negative behaviors may require 3-8 weeks of use. Dr. Bach wrote: *To conquer a fault or a wrong requires steady development of the opposing virtue (good result), not suppression.*

How are Flower Essences made?
Several flower tops, leaves, or stems are placed in distilled or purified water in a glass bowl, set in the sun for 20 minutes or up to 2 days, depending on the plant. The flower's attributes are "assigned" to the water while the sun "potentizes" the Remedy, then strained, and preserved in brandy, vinegar, or vegetable glycerin.

How will Essences help my animal?
Mental and emotional issues are addressed and re-solved. Negative behaviors are prevented from manifesting. Remedies address all facets of a difficulty, including the past, present, and the future. Behaviors change or balance again, perhaps for the first time in the animal's life. For example: develop "the virtues" of focus with Clematis, patience with Impatiens, and trust using Mimulus thus not needing to suppress the negative confusion, panic, fear or other emotional/mental obstacles and ensuring the best life possible for any animal.

Essences are successful because they address the root cause of animals' behavior problems.

How to use them?
BlackWing Farms' Remedies can be put in the drinking water, on food or treats. Sometimes, as in the case of feral or aggressive animals, just spray the remedy near them. Only 4 sprays 4 times daily for most animals. If you choose to put it in the drinking water; just add a few sprays whenever you freshen the water. Spray your hands and gently pet. Or on toys, bedding, grooming equipment, crates, stall doors, and in the bath water. Or a capful on a towel, gently apply or hang nearby— out of reach. Shared with others is fine. Guideline in homeopathy is: "Use less more often."

In Emergencies?
Use every 10 minutes for 1st hour if desired and then as necessary for calm composure & improved behavior. If they are unable to eat or drink: Put several drops on your hands and gently massage the animal. Tips of the ears is wonderful. If the animals are too far away, aggressive or unapproachable—mist the environment. DURING Hurricane Rita in Louisiana—hundreds of post-Katrina animals were calmed by misting the air. It is NOT necessary that Essences be absorbed— just get the Remedy's mist anywhere within 2-3 feet of the animals and let our Flower Essences do their work. Captured Mustangs, feral cats, trained fighting dogs and dogs used as "bait dogs" have all been successfully helped.

What about for larger animals?
Flower Essence dosage does not increase according to the size of the animal. Average is 4 drops (sprays) 4 times daily whether for a Jack Russell or a Thoroughbred or a feral cat. 2-4 sprays 6 times daily is OK too. Dosage is not about quantity but the frequency: Use less more often.

What about for very small animals?

You can use as little as 1-2 sprays twice daily and have wonderful changes occur. You be the judge. Successfully used on Birds, Fish, Pet Rats, Rabbits, Ducks, Chickens, & Iguanas.

What if other animals share the water or get some by mistake?

No problem. As a matter of fact; many people tell us the other animals improved their behavior as well. Especially in emergencies, go ahead and share!

The Good News

There is a solution for your problems no matter how chronic, ingrained, or seemingly hopeless they appear. Some special cases just take longer that's all. And yes, of course, there are the heart breakers that cannot be helped, no matter what. But we can make their last moments or days so much better with Flowers. There are some whose behavior is compromised due to physical as well as mental limitations, or actual pain. For example, King Charles Cavaliers that are having "behavioral seizures." Some of these episodes have made their way to utube videos on the internet as a source of entertainment where these dogs are growling and attacking themselves. Some spin, chasing their tails and hind legs, snapping and actually biting themselves. This severe damage can be caused by poor breeding practices from what many now call "puppy mills." In many cases, Essences will help.

Because Essences are often the last house on the block for these animals: don't give up. Expect nothing less than a miracle. Look for it. May not be what you thought but some improvement will be there. For the ones we do have to let go of—if and when that happens—then you can be assured you tried everything possible, accept that you did a good job, and go find the next one to help.

Better to Know the Truth than the Facts

Not Everything Can Be Explained. Nor should it be! Who wants to know or needs to know the exact count of stars, or the numbers of grains of sand on the beach, or the number of cells the human body has? Or the number of times our hearts will shatter from hurt and grief. Will it make a difference in the way we see the world? The way we see ourselves in the world? The way we behave? You betcha. Take away the mystery, the romance, the significance of our day-to-day lives and replace it with facts and figures and statistics—that will change us. It will change our re-actions to the World's events. Why? Because we live in and respond to the Truth of the World, not facts doled out by other humans. What I am saying here is that Truths in Nature existed long, long before scientists called them facts. And scientific facts change. Often.

Timeline of Uninterrupted Adaptation

450,000,000 years ago = first evidence of land plants.
70,000,000 years ago = first evidence of modern Felines.
60,000,000 years ago = first evidence of modern Canines.
55,000,000 years ago = first evidence of modern Equines.
100,000 years ago = first evidence of modern-day man.
60,000 years ago = first evidence of human civilization.
11,000 years ago = first evidence of domestication.

Animals behave just fine in their natural environments thriving for +/- 60 million years. Whereas, we started domesticating them for our own purposes +/- 11 thousand years ago, a blink of the evolutionary eye.

Who are you going to listen to? Perspective = we are less than a speck of dust on Earth's timeline. Give plants credit they know what they are doing after all this time and planetary upheaval, reinventing themselves several times. Credit their capabilities and while you are at it—credit bacteria, viruses, fungi, trees, flowers, and animals that they all possess intelligence and behaviors we cannot fathom... not in millions and millions of years...

Here and Now

Every plant contains an action, a purpose, a contribution to the overall well-being of all. How do they communicate their purpose? Do they yell: "Hey, over here!"? Is it daily trial and error? Is it that the animals just know? Do they know something or remember something we can't? However you slice it or ask the question, we can all agree there is something going on here on the planet and we can get a glimpse, a fascinating, glimpse. Even die-hard skeptics will be a bit more open to this opportunity when they read about Essences and also about other skeptics that succumbed. I have accepted that Essences are usually the last house on the block and my hope is that people will approach this idea before damage or injury has occurred. What's better than fixing a problem? Preventing one.

I believe with all my heart that if our intention and our purpose is to help; we will be of help. I also believe that all the information we need to be of help to others is readily available. Maybe we just need to be in the right place at the right time to see it or hear it unfold. These stories I am about to tell did not take place overnight nor were they without a cost. My purpose in telling you all this is to let you know, you are always in the right place at the right time. Always.

Making a Long Story Short
The Beginning that Lasted 20 Years

Here are some experiences never before shared—not even with my best friends, not in this detail and not with this level of honesty. I have asked myself why not and the conclusion is they would not have believed me and if they did; they would not have understood. But you will. You will because either you have been through something similar or you want to. This journey took decades to unfold. The experiences stacked on top of one another revealing a world I became comfortable in. It turns out... Actually, I have no idea how it turns out. So, guess that I too, as a willing participant, will have to wait and see.

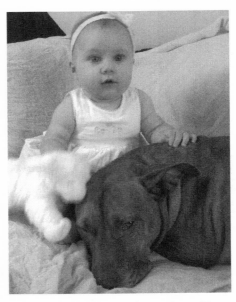

My GrandDaughter, Jade and my GrandDog, Shorty.

Mae West Started It All

Indeed, Mae West did start it all—right after she almost ended it all. Let me explain. Mae West is an American Mustang. There are rumors out there about Mustangs bonding with only one human, commonly called "a one-person horse." The day I put my foot in her stirrup; I set out to dis-prove this old wives' tale while proving my own uniqueness.

Original observations about this Mustang: she was short, shabby, aloof, and definitely not interested in anything—not her owner, not her pasture mates, and not in plodding me down the trail. With any new horse, I like fencing because it gives me a sense of security plus I don't have to walk far to get back on... just in case. However, the arena was occupied with a birthday party where wanna-be Cowgirls pushed their pink, felt hats out of their faces and climbed aboard their mighty steed, a One-Trick-Pony trotted out for such occasions. So the Mustang and I hit the trail with the actual owner behind us on another horse.

While saddling up, the owner said: "I invited you today because I want to know if Mae West will let anyone else ride her." I thought: "Fair enough."

What wasn't fair was her neglect in telling me the last person to ride Mae West, 5 years ago, was her own brother and this horse was the deciding factor in breaking his arm that day.

We had been riding for 45 minutes along a trail in Torrey Pines Park headed to the top of a bluff for a view of the Pacific Ocean. Horse people are romantics—for lack of a better word. The setting, the destination, the ambiance, and the animal all matter. So here I am riding an American icon through unique vegetation with no other humans within eyesight. At that moment of consciousness, adding to the ambiance of it all, I heard a Hawk's shrill cry. No sooner had I focused on the sky when the distance between myself and the Hawk shortened.

Most horses, at least all that I have ridden, crouch slightly before they go up. But not this Mustang. She went up. Way up. And, of course, way down. She slammed all 4 feet into the ground simultaneously and straight away, left the ground in the exact same manner. Several times as best I can recall. I rode the abrupt rhythm for several explosions knowing I would not be able to settle her and gracefully dismount.

While still thinking I had time to survive, my mind spoke to me: "If you are so in control; then why is your face 6 inches from the desert floor?"

I was a B-52 bomber without landing gear hitting face first—right side to be exact (if we ever meet; I'll show you the scars) making contact with the ground, propelled, pushed without warning and without permission a long way. I had the presence of mind that I didn't want to tumble—my head was in no position to be passed by my feet.

Being a horseperson who has been dis-lodged more than once, when I finally stopped moving, my first thought was to look for my horse. All that could be seen of Mae West was tail, dust, and the stirrup leathers slapping her sides, egging her on past her 35 mph speed limit. I knew she was going to shorten that 45 minute walk considerably and I… with the owner on another horse chasing the dust… I started walking home. Something I had done before and something I would do again.

A Cowboy and A Gentleman

Previously, I used the word: romantic. Let me say, a horseperson's idea of romance is twisted and often tied with irony. For example, resigned to walking back to the barn, I brushed off the sand and dust that would weight me down, straightened out the sunglass frame, and tilted my head up not with pride but so the blood would not drip as fast. Then, I began walking.

That's when I saw him. "HIM" was a brilliant white, gaited horse with a massive arched neck and massive white mane and there was a "HE" atop wearing an equally brilliant white shirt. No, I don't remember exactly what HE said. But I said: "No. Thank you. I'm still bleeding."

HE pulled his foot from his stirrup, leaned down, and offered me his hand. I got up behind his saddle and his Stallion glided us home. I tried to not get blood on the back of his shirt. I tried harder to figure out how I was going to get his phone number. Maybe we could go riding together some day. Hey, "HE" started it. Rode right up to me on a white horse and rescued me from a long walk home. Alas, like a lot of good men in my life, I never saw him again.

Here's another old wives' tale: Always get back on the horse that threw you."

The owner said Mae West was already back in her pasture.

The equestrienne here protested: "I have to ride her. Right away."

The owner said: "You'll frighten the children."

"What?"

"You have blood on your face."

"I'll wash it off."

"No. I mean you have a lot of blood on your face."

I rinsed my face off with a hose near the water trough and glanced down to see how the rest of me looked. My shirt was wet. And pink. It was white when I put it on this morning. Now, it was as pink as those cowgirl hats crowding the arena. I let go of the idea of re-mounting the Mustang but I did ask to go see her.

It was the third dropperful in my mouth before I asked out loud what was this she was giving me and then the horse and then me. The owner said: "Flower Essences."

"I use Flower Essences," I said.

"I use them on my horse." She said and again dispensed more liquid to me, then to the horse, more to me and then to the horse.

My Favorite Pub

Not clear on the timeline. But, I do know what happened 32 hours later in a bar. The right side of my face was now full of color and texture. Inquiries received several versions of the truth. I was testing stories. Romantic license. When I could not add up the evening's bar tab, the rugby-playing bartender commanded: "Look at me."

He said: "You have a concussion. A good one." Only then did I think of the Flower Essences and how I drove home from the barn. How did I drive home from the barn? How I napped soundly when I got home. Oh, don't start on that silly old wives' tale. OK. I should not have slept—that is true—tell everyone you know. Only then and the days following did I recognize the incredible efficacy of the Essences. Mae West was just fine, according to the owner. My untreated concussion was just fine.

Following the accident, my constant thought was: "Flower Essences for animals—what a concept." Rattling my memory as to how, where, and why I had used Flower Essences in the past, I realized those damaged alcoholic teenagers I worked with in the 1970's had the same emotional and behavioral issues as the damaged horses I encountered. These teenagers were often abused, neglected and with emotional needs left unmet by their caregivers and providers. The teenage alcoholics were scared, confused, emotionally immature, untrusting, fighting authority as well as friendships, often hurting themselves. The list goes on ad infinitum.

So the parallel shift began… From treating damaged teenagers to treating damaged animals.

Teenagers and Alcohol in the 1970'S—Mending the Person(ality)

It was not heroics nor a nobler calling that made us want to start the residential rehab facility for teenage alcoholics. We saw a need and wanted to fill it. Addiction to street drugs was being treated at a local hospital but the alcohol-craving kids coming out of or stuck in the system surrounding juvenile hall, the foster care system, etc. were not being helped in any way. Left to rot around with other criminals idling precious time away with nothing better than to exaggerate their stories of crime and passion trying to shock others. These human beings were lost to their families and into a system that could not help them.

We wanted them so we took them. My partner (in crime) and I worked for 18 months to get funding and with a staff of one and 2 halves and we opened the doors to Woodstock, a long-term, co-ed, residential treatment facility for teenage alcoholics in 1976. There was one other home-based facility addressing teenage alcoholics located on the Dine' Reservation in northern Arizona—the only other one in all of the United States.

Children coming to us were emotionally shut down, either aggressive or withdrawn, and with such a skewed outlook on life that, in the beginning, we—the "staff" were overwhelmed with worry that we were not going to be effective in turning these lives around. And to prove the point, we had runaways, suicide attempts, drug overdoses, all with defiance and mayhem.

Honestly, more times than not, we had slow progress or sometimes, none at all. One young man's progress was non-existent. He was the youngest in the house—14. His story, according to the written records of the court, was so horrific that we'd all rather have thrown the paperwork out, pretend it never happened, and start over. He had been with us 3 weeks and had not talked to anyone. We were warned by the personnel at juvenile court this could happen. Not even our "snitch" got anything from him. Nothing. Not at mealtime, not late at night, not with other residents, not with the counselor. No verbal communication, not even a phone call since he had arrived at our house with his paper bag of belongings. Nothing. Not one word.

This kid had my heart. His story had to change. Recovery was the only way that could happen. And I wanted to be there and be a part of that change. Flower Essences! Why not? Obviously, there was nothing to lose here as we had nothing to begin with here. I had been dabbling with Flower Essences for a few years. Impatiens had worked well on increasing my patience. Or so everyone else said. And Oak Essence worked well on decreasing my boyfriend's issues of depression.

So I started researching which Flower Essence Remedies would be appropriate to pull out this young man's authentic personality in a positive way. I had learned flowers made into essences worked well on rearranging the negative personality. Even to where thinking patterns are transformed. My impatience and irritation at certain events or at certain people was "tempered" when I put Impatiens Flower Essence in my drinking water or under my tongue.

But what about these kids?

What would possibly help my young favorite? Looking at the personality would tell me what to treat. My young man was quiet, depressed, shy, non-confrontational, and addicted to alcohol. From his records, we knew he was raised by his Grandparents but they were too old and too isolated on the Navajo Reservation to properly take care of this boy, his education, and meet his emotional needs. He went into the foster care system and now his story included physical abuse, drinking, and running away a lot.

It had been 3 weeks without one word from this resident. The good news was he had not tried to run away, had not fought, nor had he gotten beat up by any of the others. He showed up for meals on time and ate well. He showed up for individual and group therapy sessions but never shared one word. He watched television in the living room, never expressing pleasure or displeasure in the programming choices.

Brandy was the preservative used in Essences and thus limited me in the way I could administer a Remedy to an alcoholic. Since I believed in the power of the Essences, I decided to test it. I sprinkled them on the floor. What else could I do? I sprinkled Impatiens to increase patience, Oak for the strong, steadfast, and exhausted person, Agrimony for drawing out the true person from behind the mask, the façade of an unauthentic personality, and Star of Bethlehem for shock and victims of abuse.

Nothing. Absolutely no change the first day. The second day, I swear there was eye contact but no one was there to verify. Day 3, the staff—all 3 of us—were sitting in our office discussing the residents when the door flies open. Knocking first was a big rule. Nonetheless, our door flies open, it was my young favorite with his first words in three weeks: "Meg, The Gong Show's on TV." He closed the door and left us with stunned silence dripping off our faces. We were too shocked at his outburst to know how to respond. It seemed so rough and loud because we had strained for weeks to hear any utterance from this young man and here was an outburst. We were still staring at each other when a staff member yelled at me: "Well, what are you waiting for? Go!"

What was I supposed to do with this new responsibility? He had put the ball in my court and I had no idea what game we were playing. What I did know was this was going to be a very important 30 minutes. Do I gush all over him? Ignore him? Strike up a conversation? What? I was actually afraid being granted this unique responsibility. You know what I did? I watched the Gong Show. Without saying a word. We laughed at its silliness. He had been quiet for so long; his laughter was startling. His breakthrough was startling. I was hooked. Flower Essences had entered his silent world of hurt and gave us back a bright, artistic teenager who then started on his own road to recovery. What helped? The intention to help. Plus water, flowers, and sunshine.

Captain Morgan, the Colicky Filly, and an Epiphany

Horses are not a "convenient" animal to house and take care of even on a good day. Horses like consistency and predictability in a quiet, calm environment. Low levels of chronic stress (or a onetime traumatic situation) can have negative effects on the digestive system and the entire working system of the horse—including mental, emotional, and behavioral health.

We can, fairly easily, meet their simple demands of being equine: allow living in a herd setting in several acres with a variety of grasses and flowers to graze. Historically, in the wild, they survive by grazing on a variety of plants and grasses 12+ hours while walking 20+ miles daily.

This is how they are wired—to move, graze, and play—and how they survived and thrived for 50,000,000 years until the first humans began to restrict their freedom and feed them what was convenient.

Stress—A Horse's Enemy

From *The Tao of Equus* by Linda Kohanov:

"I told her about the [equine] enteric nervous system, how the small intestine, as a protective response, automatically becomes inflamed when the body feels threatened—even if the socially conditioned conscious mind refuses to acknowledge the threat. As a result, the small intestines of horses experiencing long-term stress remain inflamed, making them more susceptible to bouts of abdominal discomfort, or *colic*."

Captain Morgan's Story

It would be a month before I heard the black horse had a nickname: Widow Maker. He was not a popular horse. He had bucked off a lot of people. He just exploded and dumped them. I rode him a few times but he was nervous, short tempered, barely tolerating leg pressure. Unmistakably, he was ready to explode. He vet-checked sound so it was up to me to work the emotional kinks out of him. I needed to find out where the previous training had de-railed.

My first impression was he was either started too young or had an overall immature personality. The flower essences I tried on him were Impatiens for more patience with himself, his surroundings, and others; Passion Flower for comfortable correction allowing him to see the opportunity in the moment; Clematis to sharpen up his focus when I was asking something of him; and Chestnut Bud for sorting through the requests. However, within the following days, none of these made any difference to his comfort level. He was still edgy, uncomfortable, and unpredictable. This never happened to me. I was disappointed, dismayed, and nervous, asking myself, "Now what do I do?"

I gave him flower essences and homeopathic remedies for post-trauma and relaxation: Arnica essence and homeopathic 30x increasing to 200c when no bodily changes were evident. Additionally, I used

Echinacea and Yarrow essences for negative memories associated with a particular environment, also used for horses who don't like arena riding or riding on the trail away from the herd. These are the same essences and remedies I used for horses trapped and injured after a weeklong firestorm in southern California 7 years ago and also rescuing post-Katrina in 2005.

Plus I continued giving him lots of Impatiens essence as this was his biggest personality deficiency: patience with himself and others. Homeopathic Chamomila 6x was given and added to his bath water. Star Tulip for grounding was another important essence used at this time, since nothing seemed to be immediately helping.

I quit riding him until I had a definitive answer to the erratic and dangerous behavior, working him at liberty in a large 80' round pen. The new training goal was to maintain a good attitude, focusing his attention on me, waiting for my signals and meeting my requests in a timely manner. My requests were simple: Don't break gait—if trotting, stay trotting; and Don't reverse without being asked. He rebelled at my requests by striking the air several times in my direction. He picked up the pace, so I encouraged it. He did have stamina equal to his determination.

As he worked himself on the rail, I began to hear the sound of distant gunfire. He twitched his ears, slowed his pace, and looked a bit concerned. The sound got louder, more consistent. He started galloping with his hindquarters drifting just to the inside, off the rail. When the gunfire erupted again, he spooked, bucked, and kicked out a few times. This is when I realized that the gunfire was coming from him. It was gas emissions!

It had been 35 minutes including warm-up. He could go another 5-10 minutes before his cool-down period. He went 10 more minutes and he rifled out gas the entire time. Finally, he started to move more relaxed, head bowed, throat latch untroubled, belly soft and pliant, all 4 legs hitting the ground equally. His ears were actively twitching, flicking in all directions. His eyes were now more expressive, active, and blinking more often.

He had been working hard but his comfortable posture was much more than post-exercise. He had released all that build-up of painful bloat. He was darn near a puppy dog after that. I worked him several more days at liberty, let him roll as much and as often as he needed (which was a lot), made sure there was no sugar in his feed, and one day re-saddled him. His behavior improved when the gas (which had been continually replacing itself either from stress or diet) was at last eliminated. I put 2 weeks on him in the arena and on the trail riding up to 4 hours daily, without incident.

The Colicky Filly

Late one Sunday morning, my son's filly, BeauCoup StarDust, a fine Quarter Horse less than a year old, tried to colic on us. She was restless, not eating but snatching at bits of food, not drinking but walking past her bucket, pacing, pawing, had an elevated heart rate, and was looking for a place to lie down. Colic can have one or none of these symptoms and still be potentially fatal.

My flower essence remedies were closer than the phone so I gave her some flower essences mixed with appropriate homeopathic remedies. I gave her dang near everything on the shelf for relaxation, lessening the panic, limiting her pain, and getting her to eat and drink.

Then I called the vet. Actually, I called 3. The first to show up got the job. During the 90-minute wait, the filly let us spray her belly and massage her gums with flower essences of Star of Bethlehem for shock, Arnica for negative muscle memory, and Rock Rose for steadfastness, plus lightly massage pressure points including those along the Triple Heater meridian, and gently stroke her ears. You need to do what you think is right at a time like this with your horse. I walk them if possible. That day, I let her get down on her side and roll—not all the way over—but stay on one side and stretch and move her legs, getting up with a jostle and walking off immediately. Soon the young horse pushed out a piece of manure. One.

We all cheered like she'd passed the Hope Diamond.

Certainly don't want to sound like a hero here because when the filly was sick, I was truly one step, one thought away from terror. At that stage of my life, I *believed* Essences worked but, I did not *trust* them. Not with my son's horse. When our vet did arrive, she looked at the filly, watched the way she was moving, listening that she had eaten, drank and pooped. She was very pleased. My entire family was pleased. We pulled this filly through a potentially dire situation. We were getting validation from the vet. I was on a high. I crashed when she said: "That'll be $150 for the ranch call."

Wish I could tell you it was a spiritual experience, voices from beyond, something mystical that lead me from **belief** to **trust** in "home remedies" however, honestly… it was that $150. That $150 was my personal, private Scarlett O'Hara moment. Standing in the wind, face smudged with dirt, declaring: "I will never write another check for colic. Never again."

This moment could not have occurred any earlier in my life. I was 48 years old and had first successfully used Essences 25 years earlier. Here I was standing on the fence knowing I had to throw my weight, my belief, to one side or the other.

Angels did not sing and doubt still dogged my decisions during this transformative stage while I quit certain habits. Habits including choices in feed, training schedules, vaccinations, shoeing, bitting, and incorporating active prevention practices. I was well aware of these alternative choices but now I had the trust to implement them with conviction while expecting and receiving excellent results in the health and overall well-being of all the animals in my care.

BeauCoup StarDust, the filly, tried twice again to colic and these times I did not call anyone. I went straight for the same Essences. Not that I did not have my doubts and fears that my decision could end in disaster. But each time I used something "out of the ordinary" and had remarkable results; then the next time, application came with experience, resolve, and trust. Two years passed before we sold the filly and she never had another belly ache.

Decisions about protocol and procedures rests with experience, comfort levels, and a yearning to do the right thing for everyone concerned. Not easy to stand alone; but look around, there are more of us than you imagined.

Simple Changes

Make life comfortable for horses, even with changes as simple as height of feeders and waterers. Anatomically, horses are designed as grazers—always eating off the ground. Scott Haskell, DVM said, "I have $1,000 feeders so they can throw their hay on the ground and eat." We put mats down because of the sand in our area.

Encourage drinking low and long even if they have to spread their legs a touch to get that lower lip deep into the water source. Their eyes flutter, ears move, and throat latch gets soft while they enjoy a long drink. One avoidable mistake is automatic waterers. Matt Matthews, DVM, said, "Automatic waterers create a constant state of fluctuating dehydration."

The amount of time horses eat is important to them also. We had a pony whose health was compromised and we were told to feed his hay in pellet form. He wolfed down his allotment in 20 minutes. Before the week was out, he was bored, cranky, not drinking as much, and starting to exhibit nervous, stressed behaviors. We found a grass hay that his system could tolerate and also started feeding him lunch.

Try not to change feed or feeding schedules abruptly. If you buy a horse, buy a week's worth of his feed and introduce your new feed and schedule gradually. Find out what treats the previous caregivers fed and continue on with those.

Ounce of Prevention

A Cleansing Recipe for good gut health:

For 1 average adult horse; feed daily for 7 consecutive days every month. Also, some give this treat once a week.

1 cup psyllium husks—cheapest is the no-frills kind at your health food store

1 or 2 Tablespoons fresh or dried garlic

Dehydrated carrot, apple, alfalfa flower and leaves, red clover, and dandelion—available in bulk at health food stores

Mix with enough applesauce to roll and shape into bite-sized balls, then roll in more alfalfa, red clover or dandelion. Feed this daily for 1 week. Store in airtight container in refrigerator; use within 7 days. Check with your health care professional for your horse's needs.

Being Earnest

A year later, leaning over my new neighbor's fence talking horses, he questioned me about the markings on this bucking black Morgan Horse doubting it could be the same Widow Maker that had bucked off some of the best Cowboys in North County including several at his ranch.

"Yes, he was black with a white snip on his forehead. Yes, he had a piece of white above one front hoof. Yes, he was short." I answered all his questions except my clients name.

After a lengthy conversation, my Cowboy neighbor was now convinced that I had, indeed, put 30 days on the infamous Widow Maker. His parting comment to me was:

"Yes, maybe you did ride him 30 days.

But, you didn't ride him 31.

Now, did you?"

The Real Reason I Went to New Orleans was My Son's Border Collie, Chocolate Chips

I was still debating with myself about going to New Orleans where Hurricane Katrina had struck only one week earlier. Along with the rest of the nation, I watched TV as another person was rescued off another rooftop by helicopter. For days, this man refused to be rescued because there were 3 dogs on that rooftop dependant on him for food and water.

Sweltering heat burned the 3 dogs' feet during the day and this man dragged a blanket down a few steps to the flooded second floor, dipped the blanket in brackish Lake Pontchatrain water and dragged it back up to the roof. One day, he scraped against a piece of protruding metal. It was not a deep cut and did not bleed a lot. However, the next day, there were purple streaks running up his leg. That night, his leg started to swell. When the helicopter did its daily return trip to see if he was ready to leave—he flagged them down. He had to get medical attention. And there was no way the dogs could leave with him.

All I remember now from the news cast was the image of the helicopter leaving and the dogs on the roof watching it. One paced back and forth and while keeping his gaze on the aircraft. He jumped off the roof. He looked up at the helicopter and started swimming. Broke my heart. I had the same reaction September 11th when we watched, as a nation, while our hearts were breaking. It was not, could not, be real. It hurt too bad. Tears and sobs were uncontrollable. I looked for something real. Call a friend. Feed the horses. Do the laundry. But nothing was real except that dog swimming after the helicopter in the city of New Orleans.

My dogs would have done that—well 2 out of 3. But that's still good odds. What I knew in that moment: *I would want someone like me to take care of my animals if something like this had happened in my hometown.*

Just then, at that exact moment, I realized Chocolate Chips was staring at me. Just staring. Chips had those Border Collie eyes. Melted chocolate. When she looked at you, she looked straight at you and you did what you were told. Feed her, let her out, pet, play, or move whatever was in her way of her getting up on the couch.

I looked at her and said out loud: "What?"

I was wondering if she was upset by my crying. "What?"

A little exasperated: "Couch? Door? Food? What?"

She just kept staring at me, into me. Remembering my recent thought of "…take care of my animals…"

This time, I said out loud: "Should I go?"

She spoke into my heart as I heard: "You have to go. Can't you hear them crying?"

When these animals "talk" to me like this, there is no audible voice. Instead, there's a "knowing" of the words. They have been taken in. Taken somewhere within. And if it is the truth; there is a "knowing" of that too. Animals don't lie. Well, Ginaid *exaggerated* once. The red-head Quarter Horse mare told a psychic the reason she was bucking and rearing on the trail was there was a Mountain Lion and she wanted to protect us and run home. A minute later, she told the psychic there was no Lion, she just wanted to run home but didn't want to scare my 5 year old son sitting in front of me in the saddle.

Back to Katrina

I went. Everything fell into place as it does when you are truly destined to be somewhere, do something. Two weeks later, thanks to friends and family, I boarded a plane to Baton Rouge (New Orleans airport was still closed) with a new cell phone, one suitcase, and 100 pounds of natural remedies to give away.

I lied to my family when I said I had a ride from the airport with the Louisiana State vets' office. I phoned the office and the vet said "things were a little chaotic." I had served in large animal rescue for 8 years and knew if anyone used a word like chaotic—then "things" must be nuts. He was trying to figure out over the phone if I was one of the lunatics that come out for events of chaos and drama. I assured him I was a horse person and could handle my own.

"Actually, I can apply a pressure wrap to a wound, give an enema, and walk a stallion." He hesitated. I added: "All at the same time if needed." He was won over and asked why I was not there already. I looked forward to meeting him. I never did. He was not there when I arrived and I was assured by the ladies in the barn that my horse knowledge was not needed. Not the night I arrived, not the next morning, not to shovel manure, not to pick hooves, and not to walk a horse.

I asked where I could help and she said: "Maybe the dogs need people." The rest is history. Wonderful and amazing history that had it not been for the snub by the "horse people" and I ARE ONE as my Mom would say—that piece of my personal history would not have been as rich and colorful as it turned out to be. Fascinating.

Excerpts from the thank you letter I wrote after returning from the Gulf Region and published by Natural Horse Magazine, Flower Essence Society, and Animal Wellness Magazine world newsletter.

On October 11, 2005, I wrote:

I want to say "THANK YOU" from regions of my heart that did not exist just a few weeks ago. You allowed me to carry 100 pounds of natural medicines (enough to help thousands) to an area starved for emotional sensibility and mental stability.

The exhaustion in people's bodies was evident from the moment I arrived in Baton Rogue airport (New Orleans was still closed) September 21. But when I arrived in Gonzales, where the animals were being cared for, there was a renewed energy.

Volunteers FROM ALL 50 STATES were going out to New Orleans at 5:30 a.m. in their own vehicles rescuing pets that had been left alone for up to a month. Hundreds of volunteers remained behind to care for the animals previously brought in.

Volunteers would return to the Lamar-Dixon Expo Center beginning at 4:00 p.m. until 9:00 when the gates were closed. Search and rescue was becoming more acute as time was running low for the safety and health of the animals left behind. Volunteers were dropping food for some and bringing in up to 300 dogs, cats, and exotics every night for weeks and weeks.

I had the privilege to work alongside surgeons, nurses, veterinarians, MDs, mental health workers, hospital administrators, yoga teachers, college students and retirees... all up to their elbows in animal "stuff."

THEN CAME RITA.

Hundreds of volunteers were put on buses and evacuated 50 miles north—all but a skeletal crew for each of the 5 barns remained. That was my first of 6 "field promotions." How is staying behind a promotion? Several did not want to leave and were told to use permanent marker and write their social security numbers on their forearms. That is when it got very real.

Tornadoes, 70 mph wind and sideways rain. None of the 250 dogs in our barn (1 out of 5) were eating or drinking so we sprayed Remedies in the air. Soon afterward, the dogs settled, and 5 volunteers in soggy sleeping bags fell asleep on FEMA cots and slept through the worst part of Hurricane Rita and her spawned tornadoes. The next morning people from other barns—who had not slept at all—asked how we could have slept and why were our dogs were so quiet. And why were these dogs not stressed today, but instead enjoying their morning "constitutionals" and then eating breakfast.

A PRIVILEDGE TO CARE

The reunions we witnessed brought even the hardest of us to our knees, sobbing. More than not—their animals were all these people had left in their lives and for us to have the privilege to take care of them until they could be reunited was life-changing for us.

My biggest privilege was knowing there were people who believed in me and these "alternative medicines" supporting the efforts to carry these products to an area so desperately in need. Family and friend's donations were amazing. Kerry, Jennifer, Linda, Rachel, and Johanna worked for hours on my back porch making Remedies, bagging different proportions of 28 whole herbs in a "re-build blend" for the horses, and mixing bottles of Lavender essential oil with Remedies for the people in the region living in evacuation centers and for the volunteers exhausted by "seeing and feeling" too much.

The Humane Society of the United States made me an offer to go back and assist in the re-building of the New Orleans animal shelter destroyed by Katrina. I will fly in for a meeting within the next few weeks and see where it goes from there.

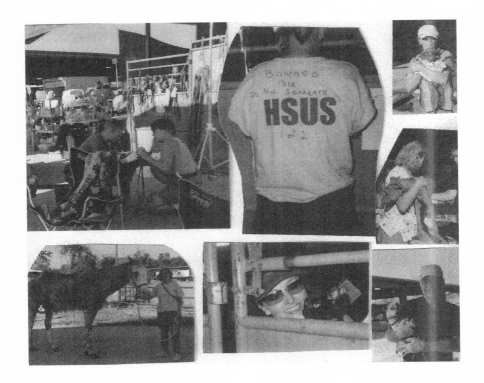

I got the job

The way I got it is not pretty.

I went to New Orleans to interview with the staff at the Louisiana SPCA. No one had any idea what that job would be, the job of rebuilding. I knew it would be emotional. But not even my imagination could fathom the depth of emotion. I got the job because I had made myself a deal. The deal was I would—to a degree—turn off "my gifts" for a while. I had to since the death and destruction, the pain and the loss, would certainly overwhelm me and I would be of no use to anyone if I succumbed to the pain. So my "in-sight" took a hiatus. Never more thankful for that than the day I got the job at the shelter.

Feral cats plus injured, sick domestics inevitably had to be euthanized. No one wanted to do it. Lists were altered. Delays were further delayed. Individual employees begged for a few more days to find homes. Problem was there were no homes. There were no more foster homes available. Everyone was maxed out and could do no more. So cats were scheduled for euthanasia. The air in the kennel area was grim that day. I was the outsider. No one knew what I was capable of so, they told me to answer the phone. It didn't ring for hours.

Screaming started. Dogs were fighting. Only one was fighting while the other was an immediate victim. The kennel's wire panels were lifted a few inches off the floor and one dog had gotten hold of his neighbor's paw. Injuries were so severe that the victim needed to be euthanized. After a procedural review by the staff; the bully was determined too aggressive to keep. All while I'm on stupid phone duty. Don't they know who I am? What I could do? Why was I here? My ego and emotions were running the full gamut.

Every animal and every person was beyond upset. Understandably. Now they had one emergency surgery with dire results, 2 dog euthanasias, lots of paperwork plus the scheduled cat euthanasias that had to take place today. I offered to help. I was told I could not. I hung around in the vet area long enough to understand that the man who could perform the euthanasias had to, wanted to, immediately assist the victim dog—she was his priority. I offered to assist with the cats.

"You can't."

"Why not?"

No answer.

I said: "I can. I can do this."

Giving in to my stubbornness, the caregiver trusted a stranger to be kind. To be as compassionate as he would be. He watched me talk softly to the cats. Reassuringly stroking the domestics and easing the discomfort in the ferals. He watched for a while. I got the job staying for 4 more months helping.

I met him.

The man in the helicopter.

The man on the rooftop with the 3 dogs.

Turns out they were not even his dogs.

His neighbors evacuated and he took care of the dogs on the rooftop. The man showed up months later at the Louisiana shelter where I was working. He wanted to feed or walk dogs. He needed the contact. He said he was not ready before but, now, he needed to be with some dogs. It was difficult to explain that the shelter was not yet open to the public.

His heart was broken.

Only a dog could help.

We understood when he left.

Liars and Thieves: Rescuers at Katrina

I met some extraordinary people, heroes no one would ever hear of—some names even I can't remember, but they were heroes. And I want to tell their stories. They were present when there was catastrophe or when there were tears to shed that would bring back health. They were there when the floodwaters rose while they took all the strays they could find and continued to feed them even when their own food was scarce.

This is where I will begin to talk of heroes: Louisiana 4 weeks after Hurricane Katrina hit the Gulf region and Lake Pontchatrain flooded the majority of New Orleans. An official asked me, a volunteer, to accompany the man and wife and give them some of the donated dog food and a few leashes and collars.

These 2 had the same hollow eyes—eyes that had seen so deeply into despair that they could not do that again and survive. So, they raised the level at which they viewed life as if that would protect them from hurting that deeply ever again.

LIARS AND THEIVES

The man waiting for his flight home had those eyes. He could not focus on, let alone eat, the food in front of him though he looked emaciated. He could not take in what was on the TV. He stared at it but just off to one side. He wanted to talk about what he had seen, talk about the lies he had told. Talk about the people, the children, the elders he saw stuck up on their roofs for days.

He had to tell me he lied when he told these rooftop survivors he had seen their neighbors, their loved ones, their family members safe and out of the flood waters.

He lied because it was the right thing to do. He lied when he told people he would be right back for them. He lied to some when he told them everything was going to be alright. No one in this ordeal was ever going to be alright ever again. Never again.

He told me he got to New Orleans early—only one day after the flooding and first off stole a boat. For weeks, he heard screams, told lies, helped the injured and frightened, told more lies and was joined in his efforts to rescue and give comfort by other liars and thieves. He saved lives. Lots of them. It cost him a piece of his own, part of an innocence never to be reversed or rest again in naiveté.

I had just arrived. I don't know how it happened but I found myself handing over my only vial of Flower Essences with Cinnamon leaf oil that was to be for my nightmares I knew would inevitably come. He took my vial, knowing it was my only one and said: "You had to give this to me. I cannot sleep. I cannot get the images, the faces, the sounds to leave. I am haunted now. Haunted by their voices, the yelling in absolute darkness. The darkness of water in the dead of night."

He clutched the vial with a promise of relief. He reached into his front pocket and pulled out a string of brown beads and said: "You had to give me this bottle. I am a Medicine Man from northern Michigan. I can't be like this." I never got his name and I never saw him again.

<u>ONE WEEK AFTER ARRIVING</u>

This man and wife, survivors with hollow eyes, standing in front of me—told me they could see dogs come out of the woods at night near their tent but any noise sent them running. So these people figured they could start feeding them to lure them out and befriend them so they would not get hurt or impounded. I asked where they were camping and all he said was: "Nearby."

They told me they had to borrow the tent and blankets. They drove a beautiful truck so I did not think they were destitute. As we loaded their truck with the scant supplies I was authorized to give, she told me they were childhood sweethearts together for 40 years and had never in their lives lived further than 5 miles from one neighborhood in the 9th Ward, both born at the local hospital 55 years ago.

While not able to or willing to form complete sentences, she said: "The storm took it all. Everything. There is nothing there now. Nothing." She scraped at the asphalt we were standing on and said: "This is what it's like now. Our neighborhood. We didn't think the storm would be this bad. Never has been before. We left for Camille but nothing since then. Who knew?"

"We were on top of our roof and no one came. The water was so fast. It took our friends' baby right out of her arms. Swept her away. There was nothing anybody could have done. But she'll never believe that. Hell, I don't even believe that."

"What I do know is that we can't go home. There is no home. There is no 9th Ward. It's gone. It's all gone."

The man looked at me through quivering eyes. Eyes that should not have seen any of this. A kind man, very gentle. He had been strong for his wife, giving her hope that everything was going to be OK.

"It's been a month and I still cry my heart out every day but he keeps it all bottled up inside." she said.

When I looked into her husband's eyes again, he must have seen something safe in mine, and he started to cry. He had held it all in to be brave for his wife and now that loss came flooding out in tears, sobs. Unstoppable. He fell into my arms and cried for a long time, no shame, no embarrassment. We were lost in the moment and when I finally looked over his shoulder for his wife, she took a step backwards and whispered: "Thank you. Thank you so much." Then, she looked at the ground and waited.

I'd been allocated to give them one bag of kibble and a few collars and leashes. By the time they drove off, they had 10 huge bags of kibble, 4 cases of canned food, dozens of collars and leashes of all sizes, several large kennels, 10 crates, yards of fencing, bags of treats, medical supplies, and relief. I had just crossed over to the world of liars and thieves.

Tex, Ginaid, and One Dollar

The first animal to talk to me made me cry. The second one made me laugh.

The first animal was a horse, a mare to be exact, named Ginaid. She came to us from an auction and now, for the life of me, I can't recall if we gave her the name or she came with it. But she was Ginaid, a red-head with an attitude. Her feet were what I was told were called Genie feet. They were so long they curled up at the ends like Genie slippers. An average hoof is 5 inches, hers were 12" and melted to a curly point. She had two thin iron shoes still attached by a few nails; both were on the left side front and back. She had to slide them along as her hooves would not roll over in the front. Indentations marked her body where a saddle must have sat for a long time, her legs were swollen, and the corners of her mouth were calloused from harsh hands on the bridle.

Her personality was aloof. Always stood by herself in the pasture and ran the others away with a turn of her head. She was last to show up at feeding time but always got the pile of hay she wanted. I waited for her to come around and befriend me. She never did. Years later, she proved she loved my young son with a ferocity that only a red-headed mother could display.

ONE CHORE

We rescued several horses that summer but paid dearly for the privilege. One 9 year old gelding had not been out of an 8' by 8' pipe corral in years. He was 6' long. Not trained and afraid of everything. The afternoon he arrived, we let him loose in his own one acre pasture and he started running. I do not mean frolicking and amusing himself. I mean running full board for hours. By 9:00 that night, I had to call Tex and ask if the horse was going to be OK. All he could say was: "Well, at least the horse is not going to colic. Not tonight anyways."

One other animal in my life did the exact same thing. She was a Border Collie named Bear. We rescued her from our local humane society. They held on to her for 11 months. Against all rules. Don't tell anybody but I am pretty sure they moved her around, changed her name a few times and often "lost" her paperwork. She was that same fantastic black and white with soft, functional fur and doe brown eyes that pierce right through to your heart and soul. A dog you can trust.

Bear was adopted by my 7 year old son because we had lost our well-loved 14 year old Border Collie, Jade. Elegant and authentic. Jade died in my arms while I slept. No other dog has ever given me a greater parting gift. I will have more of her story later on. Like the time she got bit by a dinosaur while playing with my young son.

Here I just want to say that Bear Dog too ran and ran when she got to our place. The Border Collie lived in a cage for almost a year and needed to log a lot of miles.

Back to Ginaid and the conversation I did not know was going to happen.

Calendar-wise we were somewhere around 1990. My son was 3. We moved to the country. As my friend would describe it: "We aren't in the middle of nowhere. We are 8 miles from the middle of nowhere." Some even described it as backcountry. I liked that. What had happened to bring about the move was when I told my 3 year old to feed his beloved Jade. He torted: "I don't have to."

Time froze. He had one chore to do and he was refusing to do it—take care of his only pet. I vowed with my best Scarlett O'Hara voice that we would live in a land where there were lots of chores. Within a few months we moved from a lovely beach community with lovely houses in a lovely neighborhood with a single chore to living on 40 dusty acres with lots and lots and lots of chores. So many chores I almost called it work. Did Mike keep his one chore? I don't remember. There was so much work it all blurred together.

THE HORSES

We were going to buy, ride, and then sell horses we would find cheap and sell expensive. Anyone know the horse business? Old adage is still true: To make a million dollars in the horse business you start with two million and only lose one.

My "partner" Tex picked out the horses and had them shipped to the house. He ignored my questions about his choices and the horses continued to show up. $700 here. $1,000 there. Not trained. Not healthy. One had a really big head. One was lame. One bucked me off every day. And one was old. Very old.

There were all kinds of surprises: vet bills, new equipment, tack, expensive feed, and several trips to the Osteopath for my "involuntary dismounts." One surprise was the horse named Dollar. Tex said the gelding's name was Dollar because that's what he paid for him. Tex was old and so was his horse. Tex added 30 years to his own age claiming to be 103, wore shirts with different initials and used pay phones a lot—but that is fodder for another book entirely.

Dollar was truly old. His back swayed, he walked and trotted stiff-legged, never ran, and his hair was falling out in patches. But he loved our kids and they could climb all over and under him anytime they wanted or needed. One morning, several weeks after his arrival, I realized Dollar had not eaten his breakfast. I called Tex who told me from 20 miles away that Dollar was sick. I told him that was impossible since there were no signs of it. When I turned around, Dollar was lying on the ground.

Hours of heroic efforts did not change the course of this horse's life. We were assured by the vet's tests that Dollar would not live to midnight and the last hours would be excruciating pain. We did what we believed to be the right thing.

It was sad on every level. Dollar was such a cool horse. He loved our children. He got along with everyone. He was a gentleman. And Tex loved him. He rescued him from a cruel man who had many horses and loved none of them. Our kids got to hang out with a truly good horse. And Dollar got to die with people who loved him deeply. He won all our hearts within this short time.

I sobbed. I cried for him. For the pony of my youth. For my dogs. For my parents. I sobbed. It was good, cathartic. We all cried.

A few days after we put him to sleep, I went to check on the horses after dark as was my custom. I always went alone and sometimes just hung out after checking the water levels in the troughs. This night, Ginaid walked up. Her feet had been trimmed, the swelling in her legs reduced, eating good food, and definitely settling into her position as Alpha Mare. She was still aloof and still did not care much for me. But here she was, approaching me for the first time. I had been crying so hard I did not hear her coming. I sat as still as I could while she came close to get a drink of water.

At that exact moment, I had just been thinking: This passing was very upsetting. The children were still crying off and on. I was upset. Tex was sad. Why did Dollar have to die here?

I heard: "You want to know why he died here?"

I was dumbfounded.

I heard: "Because if he would have died at his old place; nobody would have cried."

She finished drinking and walked away.

The Second One

I had just finished reading Marlo Morgan's 1990 book: *Mutant Message Down Under*. Controversial still, but one hell of a read. I was crying. Indigenous People using songlines to travel, plants to sustain and heal, communicating without words and acknowledging that all this was learned from the animals and plants of earth. And what is the future of these spiritually connected people? According to the book, it is to become extinct before all other humans.

What do I do when I am crying or upset? I go to find the horses. So here I am crying in the pasture hugging my son's Pony named: Pony Bologna. Still crying, I say out loud: Do you guys really communicate without sounds?

"Do you see my lips flapping?"

I heard it. In my head. In the air. Somewhere. But, I heard it.

I had not tried to communicate with Ginaid or anyone else with fur and hooves since that night by the water trough. To tell the truth, it kind of freaked me out. Obviously, it really freaked me out. Otherwise, I would have tried to communicate again or at least, told someone about the experience. I did not. I ignored it. Chalked it up to a vivid imagination. Even though her words that night had greatly comforted me, I told no one.

So, now, here is Pony Bologna clearly asking me a question.

I said: "What did you say?"

I hear: "You heard me the first time. I am not going to repeat myself."

This can't be happening.

I hear: "I know you heard me."

I said: "Well, do you?"

I walked back to the house just ahead of his echo accentuating a different word each time: "**Do** you see my lips flapping? Do **you** see my lips flapping? Do you **see** my lips flapping?"

Pee Cups

There was an article in a 2005 San Diego newspaper, written more for amusement than reporting, about an event so extraordinary that the dialogue it started in my house would change my world forever. The article was about an OB/GYN who brought home Dixie cups full of urine. I am saying what I read not necessarily what was written. I'm sure he used professional specimen jars. As I was saying, the doctor brought home several Dixie cups full of urine from healthy patients and one from a patient who had been positively diagnosed with cancer.

The doctor set up these cups of urine, spaced several yards apart, and allowed his dog, his innocent and uneducated, 30 pound mutt, to enter the room. The dog sniffed the cups of urine and sat down by the one belonging to the woman with cancer. Just sat and waited.

No. He had no training for detection. He had no commands from his "person." Was Lassie trained to run back the house, spinning and barking every time someone fell in the well? I don't think so.

Forgive me if you think I am making light of this and especially of cancer. I am not. But what I am saying is we are surrounded by an intelligence so far superior to ours that I am constantly in shock and awe every single time we can document an event like what happened to this mutt and his person, the cancer cells and the olfactory system of a canine. I'm sure that doctor was never quite the same.

Now, I am thinking: "Why this dog? What's so special about this mutt that he can detect cancer from pee cups."

"We can all do that."

Chocolate Chips, my son's Border Collie, was the only breathing being in the room. My first reaction was to start imitating Robert DeNiro out of nervous fear with tough talk: *Hey, you talkin' tu me?*

Instead, I get cocky and sass: "Then, why don't you *ALL* help out like this dog?"

"Because (audible sigh) no one asks."

The Power of Possible

Every single thing
you see as matter
and know as fact
used to be invisible.
Every single thing.
Invisible.
And there's lots more
where that came from.

Why are we here?

To prove my theory about the efficacy of Essences or to sufficiently piss you off so you will set out to prove me wrong and while in that process, fall in love with the power of Essences—because that is inevitably where that road leads.

In reality, we are here because we have 30 minutes to save a life. Tick tock…

Seriously, problematic behavior is always the #1 reason for euthanasia of healthy animals. Does not matter what other names they attach like landlord dispute, barking when not home, or an incontinent cat—it is behavior. There are dismal statistics of avoidable euthanasia, injuries, and harm to humans.

Here is my theory, premise, and promise to you:

Flower Essence Remedies Improve Behavior.

Flower: peak of highest development, crowning achievement, the highest example or best representative of something.

Essence: the intrinsic or indispensable properties of a thing.

Remedies: therapies that relieve pain or correct a disorder. For our purposes, we are always referring to emotional and mental "pain."

Improve: to make better or become better.

Behavior: anything that an organism does involving Action, Re-action, Response to its environment or stimulation. (2) The ability to survive in existing environment. (3) A mentally guided emotion, action, or re-action.

While proving this theory, I will lay out some facts of incredible actions and behaviors that exist right here, right now. My intention is to broaden your curiosity about the collaborative experience of our world's inhabitants. My purpose is to make it meaningful, improving your life and those you love and care for.

The Simple Truth is Not Complicated

The 2004 Tsunami killed more than 240,000 people yet not one animal died. Not one. A story from that day says a lot. Fishermen, headed back into Puket Island, Thailand, with a full boat of fish noticed the dolphins that should be following their boat for a free meal, were actually swimming back out to sea. This unusual behavior caused the fishermen to "listen" to the Dolphins and turn their boat around. When they did this, there was nothing unusual at all about the weather or the waves, but without apology, they followed the Dolphins back out toward open sea. When they turned to look; the first tsunami wave hit the shore. It must have been underneath the boat when they followed the Dolphins' lead. Villagers in the devastated areas said the Elephants started retreating to higher ground days before the Tsunami hit. Dogs and Cats not tethered (unlike the 2005 floodwaters of New Orleans) were also spared.

Toxoplasma is a brain parasite that lives and thrives in cat feces. This is the reason expectant mothers should not clean litter boxes nor be close as no one has proven this parasite cannot be inhaled. And in my opinion, cats should not sit on laps during pregnancy—erring on the side of caution. During laboratory experiments in Europe, when the research mice were injected with Toxoplasma, these mice were no longer afraid of cats. NOT AT ALL. The parasite had overtaken the natural instinct "telling" them not to be afraid of their predator. The parasite took this host hostage to act out ITS own survival.

Rabid Animals (Dogs, Fox, Coyote, Skunks, Raccoons, Bats, while low risk carriers include Rats, Mice, Opossums) act aggressive and bite because the Rabies Virus is in control of the animals' behavior causing aggression in even the most friendly pet. Rabies virus is in the saliva and injected by the "hypodermic" teeth straight into the bloodstream of its "next host." The virus is clearly in control of ITS own destiny creating "abnormal" behavior in its unsuspecting host.

Pulitzer prize winning author, Jared Diamond in his fascinating 1997 book, *Guns, Germs, and Steel,* puts it best, writing: "For modification of a host's behavior, nothing matches rabies virus, which not only gets into the saliva of an infected dog but drives the dog into a frenzy of biting and thus infecting many new victims."

Looking back when I was growing up in Illinois, we saw rabies in a few wild animals and even one dog. What I remember is their behavior was friendly at first, meaning they would approach closer than a "normal" wild animal and that would tip off my Mother that this animal was not "in its right mind." Sure enough, when they approached with this stealth, they would get close enough you could see the drool and foam FULL OF VIRUS prior to attacking and biting.

Influenza virus has 8 DNA markers or genomes as they are called. Humans have 25,000 DNA markers. The flu virus killed twenty million people in 1918-1919 worldwide and continues to kill up to 500,000 people worldwide every year. How does it persist against our vast 25,000 genomes? By making our bodies behave in a way that will spread the virus, simply coughing and sneezing on our families, friends, and neighbors. Watch someone sneeze or cough into their hands and then follow them for a few minutes and see what, who and how that one person infects others thus proliferating the virus. Soap, disinfectant, or sunshine kills the flu virus. These 25,000 genomes just need to remember to: WASH YOUR HANDS.

The Truth of the Matter is You Can't Make This S_it Up

One clever virus has been documented wearing an overcoat made entirely of bacteria, pulling it over itself like a cape and travels undetected through the body. If anything is found to be out of balance or causing harm, the bacteria is attacked and killed, leaving the virus free to find another disguise.

Bacteria, collectively and singularly, is the coolest thing ever. Wait until you hear about *Halobacterium Salinarum*. It's an amazing story. Back in the 1930's, someone in northern Michigan wanted to tan an animal hide with salt and sunshine. He remembered seeing salt crystals while exploring a cave. He gathers the salt, spreads the crystals on the hide and sets it in the sun. Bacteria formed on the hide which should not happen. The scientists of the day could not identify the bacteria since it did not "exist" (yet). Not until the 1970's was there an explanation. Turns out this cave was formed when the salt water sea receded during a climate change dating back 419,000,000 years and left behind salt deposits containing *Halobacterium Salinarum*.

When the bacteria was brought out of the cave and set on a moist hide in the sunshine—IT RE-POPULATED. That's the word the scientists use, not me. THE BACTERIA RE-POPULATED, as in CAME BACK TO LIFE after FOUR HUNDRED and NINETEEN MILLION YEARS.

Know what else "re-populates"? Fleas. As in household Cats' and Dogs' fleas.

Flea eggs, possibly carrying the bacterial infection caused by *Yesinia pestis* responsible for creating bubonic plague, live up to 7 years and RE-POPULATE under the right conditions. These 3 simple conditions are a moderate temperature, vibration, and carbon dioxide. That's it. What that means is, a human (or an animal), walks into a house (moderate temperature) where the eggs have waited up to 7 years (walking creates suitable vibration) and breaths (exhaling carbon dioxide). If any of these new fleas is infected and bites someone; bubonic plague is injected straight into the bloodstream, assuring the plague's survival.

Coincidence: to happen at the same time or occupy the same place simultaneously, in our discussion, like a problem and its remedy.

Gypsies in the Palace. During the Bubonic Plague pandemic which killed 30-35% of the European population in the 1300's, Gypsies were said to be able to rob the dead victims without getting sick themselves or spreading the Plague to others. It is also said Gypsies were "greasy." Particular plant oils combat bacterial infections. Oils purportedly used by the Gypsies included: Cinnamon, Cloves, Rosemary, Lemon and/or Lemongrass, and Tree leaves—coincidentally growing exactly where needed to keep people safe and healthy.

Malaria is a parasite using the bite of a mosquito to inject itself directly into the bloodstream. Cinchona trees contain quinine which prevents and "cures" Malaria and, coincidentally, the trees grows where Malaria thrives. Is it possible we could discuss cholera, typhoid, syphilis, MRSA, and cancer with a curiosity about respective characteristics (behaviors) of the problem and simultaneously, coincidentally see its remedy? These all have behaviors that keep themselves alive and thriving, often mutating to elude detection and destruction. So what? Well, what if...? What if you were in trouble and the help you needed was right there next to you? This is exactly what happened when building the Panama Canal where French and American workers were dying by the thousands from Malaria but, not the Panamanians. One doctor had his "aha moment" when he saw a healthy Panamanian chewing on Cinchona tree bark! The rest is history. Homeopathic history.

Every Plant Contains an Action, a Behavior, and a Personality

Every action, behavior contains a benefit, holds a value for survival... for something, with or without any prior written approval and plausible explanation. Why should you believe it? You don't have to believe anything for this to take place. This idea does not need permission to be effective since plants have been acting on the behalf of animals for millions of years without your OK. What we have done domesticating these animals, keeping them at our sides so to speak, is denied them access to what keeps them healthy and happy as the case may be. Essences can bring them the help they need to function better. That's all. This is not rocket science nor brain surgery and should not be treated as such—Flower Essence Therapy, as introduced by Dr. Bach, was always intended for the lay person, no one was to be excluded from the rewards of this practice.

THE MIND (OR THE BODY) RECOGNIZES THE NEED TO SEEK OUT (BENEFITS FROM) SPECIFIC PLANTS CHOSEN FOR ITS SPECIFIC NEEDS AND FUNCTIONS.

Nutrition is Often Available in Your Own Neighborhood

What would our domesticated animals run to if free? Probably to plants, grasses, weeds, and leaves to eat, rub against, or roll in. Animals seek out the assistance of plants, weeds, and trees before and after conception, birthing, lactating, bleeding, hibernation, treating aches, pains, worms, fungus, bacterial infections. And no, these plants are not hiding in exotic lands, unattainable and not needed in quantities that decimate its own population. And not needed for long periods of time, only when flowering, naturally dried, or easily stored. Again, please, don't pick up the phone with a plan to yell at me. This is from information I have gathered over the years and let swill around my mind, waiting to prove, disprove, argue, whatever it takes for me to write one complete sentence.

When an animal receives nourishment, the body and mind obviously recognizes the benefits and reacts appositely (implies a traceable significant logical connection.) I'm just saying... Why did my 2 horribly sick horses with E Coli accept herbs and tree bark from my hands gobbling them up like candy treats when the healthy horse next to them blew it out of my hands like it was poison? Both my horses fully recovered on this combo whereas $1,500 and 3 weeks of antibiotics had failed. My vet later called me for the recipe.

Or when my Welsh-Arab Pony of the 1960's was monthly offered tobacco unrolled from my Dad's Pall Mall cigarettes to treat for worms and ate it like sweet feed for 4-5 days. But on day 6, blew it out of my hand with a snort refusing to eat any of it. My Mom suggested creek mud for leg swelling and injuries. Spider webs to stop bleeding. After excess exercise, rub downs with left-over salt blocks crumbled inside old gunny sacks worked to prevent sore muscles. Best therapy for an athlete? A swim in salt water. When this mare retired at the age of 32, the new owners had to raise her fencing to 6' because she kept jumping out to eat fresh grass. Why? Because she could.

Emotional Nutrition Provided by Plants

Evidence proves this Animal-Plant "Conspiracy" "Collaborative Experience" "Invisible and Intelligent Behavior" is going on right in front of our eyes. In a good, good way. And for a long, long time. Plants recognize and understand the need to grow where, when, and how (Giraffes' food is up high while Badger food is not) in order to be of maximum benefit to themselves and others. Without a doubt, this is a conspiracy, replete with a wink, nod, and secret handshake working and acting together for the better good of all.

Conspiracy, coincidence, or an ancient agreement, call it what you may; watch what happens when you bring these powerful entities of plant Essences and Animals together. What occurs is the visible evidence, physical proof—demonstrated as improved behavior—of a mysterious collaborative experience that is presently going on right under our noses and most likely has been going on for a long, long time. How long? Refer to the timeline.

Again, why are we here?

To improve behavior = *the ability to survive in existing situation* (not necessarily the ideal situation) and to show you the power of what is possible while we connect the dots for animals and plants helping humans. We are here to learn how to reset "normal" behavior, thinking, patterns of learning thus creating healthy actions. Following are case studies of some of my friends and acquaintances in horrendous situations, "not in their right minds," behaving poorly, many headed for euthanasia, or serious injury.

In the Simplicity of Nature and Its Plants is the Complexity of Action. Let me explain...

So What and Who Cares?

What are Flower Essences?

Remedies created from organic material, such as flowers or leaves, placed in water, set in the sun, strained, and then offered to animals.

What do they do?

Flower Essences balance, maintain and/or repair emotional and mental health in any animal improving problematic behaviors, attitudes, emotions, and patterns of learning permanently. Essences are simple, effective, and **highly successful because they address the root cause of mental and emotional problems, not suppressing or masking the problematic behaviors to resurface later or manifest as another problem.**

Solutions to behavioral problems are available even if manifested as a physical or mental illness. For example, damage from in-line breeding practices evident in "puppy mill" animals, horses used for sport and entertainment, or feral cats. With dedication and genuine commitment to righting a wrong; debilitating conditions can often be mended.

Why use them?

Prevent and/or to reverse problematic behaviors whether puppy mill dogs, feral cats or crazy horses, no matter how long ago the problems started. Flower Essences go to the root cause of negative and unhealthy behaviors transforming problematic attitudes, emotions, and patterns of learning allowing any animal to excel to their fullest potential. Essences address situations and challenges facing domesticated animals. Not just achieving success on obvious behavioral or emotional situations but, offering long-term, permanent solutions to even chronic problems. Whether you are dealing with an excessive personality trait, an ingrained fear or a brand new experience; Remedies can give you that moment of opportunity to make IT work. Whatever your IT is at the time.

PHILOSOPHY

"The action of these remedies is to flood our natures with the particular virtue (good result) we need, and wash out from us the fault that is causing them. To conquer a fault or a wrong requires steady development of the opposing virtue*…not suppression," wrote Dr. Edward Bach, 1930's British physician.

Richard Gerber, M.D., *Practical Guide to Vibrational Medicine* calls this "emotional-rebalancing therapy." "rebalance disturbed emotional and mental patterns." These behaviors can range from depression, failure to thrive, separation-anxiety, grief, shock, fears and phobias that may lead to an animal's poor behavior. No matter whether born with the emotional/mental deficiency or resultant from exposure to stress or trauma.

Effective, permanent improvement with POSITIVE side effects.

Answers to problems faced by domesticated animals no matter what the problem, behavior, situation, or circumstance is what I am after and what I have gotten from using Flower Essences for nearly 40 years. Most answers lie in bridging the gap between an animal and its confined environment. If we can't get them free running in the woods and grasslands allowing access to their emotional nutrition—you can bring it to them in the simplest form possible: Essences.

There is no substitute for patience, positive training, and understanding but sometimes we simply need to pull the lamp closer to get a better look at the cause of the discontent. Essences will allow you to illuminate, see from a different angle, presenting the opportunity to reflect on the animals' specific needs and effect a permanent change.

Why should you believe me?

Believe the animals. There is no placebo effect in their world. Believe other people's documented magic. Tap into a source of intelligence that can't be seen, measured, weighed, dissected, or analyzed—proof is in a happy animal... Measure that.

Homeopathy Made Simple

A plant causes the same symptoms (in a healthy person) that it "cures" (in a person exhibiting those same "unhealthy" symptoms.) Homeopathic medicine addresses the root cause of a dis-ease or disorder in the overall system while allopathic medicine aims to eliminate the symptoms. I am going to leave the room now while you argue amongst yourselves.

Dr. Bach began searching Nature for a safe, gentle, non-invasive method to prevent and treat disease in humans when on his lengthy English-Welsh walk-about. He discovered that he felt emotional symptoms in the presence of certain flowers. Furthermore, if he drank the dew gathered at dawn, for one example, from the Mustard plant; he then felt depressed. (Mustard is used for lingering depression.) But when he made a Mustard Essence; the symptoms, in an already depressed person, were alleviated. Bach documented 38 remedies which included one water source and one blending of five flowers. Since then, thousands of remedies worldwide have been documented for use in humans and animals—documented but not necessarily proven effective.

In my non-anthropomorphic opinion, animals are not emotionally complicated and do not require inaccessible and exotic plants for their well-being. Without human interference of domestication and captivity, the environment where the animals naturally reside or roam provide for all animals' needs. Simple examples are vegetation available for Bears before and after hibernation. Tree barks for Deer in the dead of winter. Monkeys in need of dewormers and anti-fungals gather and ingest certain local plants at certain times of the year. Some plants are masticated and then rubbed into the fur for ticks and bugs. Goats, horses, and livestock in need of springtime cleansing or hormone balancing will find the appropriate plants readily available when needed, again barring human interference. Plants are close at hand to facilitate overall health, conception, pregnancy, during childbirth, afterbirth, lactation, etc.

Whether coincidence or by design, plants provide for all our carbon-based needs in one way or another.

Who Cares?

After years of working with rescued and "damaged" animals (and errant teenagers) headed to their end because of bad behavior; I came to believe these animals (and adolescents) were, to varying degrees, in a state of shock. Many were so surprised by their inhumane and confusing treatment that they either became aggressive, enraged, depressed, or stubborn making them unpredictable and dangerous to others or themselves.

Following the use of Essences, dramatic behavior improvements took place that seemed impossible considering the history of the animal or the circumstances, which today includes surviving hurricanes, week-long firestorms, tornadoes, and court ordered animal seizures, including hoarders. Their positive behaviors appeared no less than miraculous. You can actually see a "PAUSE" allowing the animal to make a new, positive decision whereas there was nothing but immediate, reactive, and negative behavior only minutes earlier. Essences address the current trauma and equally as important, address the past by replacing old, negative memories with healthy, positive thoughts creating all-around good results. This change affords the opportunity to learn, to accept, to cooperate with, and trust human intervention and companionship. Essences re-set normal.

Why Blends of Single Remedies? Answer: Collaboration.

Similar to companion plants improving a garden's vitality, each Flower Essence contributes to the completed process of behavior change. Blending different Flower Essences addresses the cause of dis-comfort, dis-connectedness, and dis-content resolving any resultant troublesome behaviors while establishing the reality of a new, positive experience. For many animals, accomplishing permanent behavior change requires a multi-faceted process requiring more than one Flower. Essences address not just the symptoms but the feelings and past bad results so that the entire experience can now be affected, influenced positively.

Imagine your animal's life as a set of blueprints.

The master plan reflects how the foundation, structure, circuitry, plumbing, and mechanics must work together to achieve success. If part of the plan is missing or out of sync, then all symmetry is lost and results are potentially disastrous. Synchronizing your animal's blueprints to reflect its master plan results in the success of the entire venture.

Focusing on the outcome, each Flower brings out the best in the others while working together to create a positive behavior change. Eliminating the negative effects on the personality helps acquire long-term resolution ensuring optimum decision-making and positive behavior in the future. New experiences are softened, accepted, and made into gentle life experiences. ...*always building on the steady development of good.*

Essences succeed due to the fact they deal with the root cause of the problem and literally or figuratively, re-write the experience of past negative experiences and its resultant un-healthy behavior.

Be willing to go the distance and see where the animal leads you.

Maybe you have mapped out the life of a Grand Prix level Dressage horse and they have the heart to jump. Or the agility dog has four front paws. Or the cat you got for little Tommy is afraid of children. Forcing our will against the animal's instincts will not lead to any level of success. Equipment and techniques are available to force the animal to do our will, but here with Flower Essences you seek the opposite. Remember,"...steady development of the opposing virtue" will always result in success. Use the correct Remedy and the sought-after resolution will become a living part of the animal. This inner-learning and acceptance will last a lifetime.

Flower Essences, using the same amount of drops for each will work for feral cats, captured Mustangs and young Jack Russells. What do you have to lose? You might have to wait a few hours, days, or weeks to see the new positive behavior. Be patient and notice the subtleties. Notice the "TRIES" your animal is giving you. Get the behavior you are seeking, knowing it is permanent, and move on to enjoy your companion.

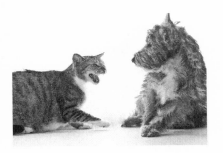

Every Body
is an

Emotional
Storage Unit

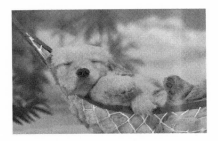

When the door to the storage unit, basement, attic opens up and light hits dark; memories slog back, and for a moment, you forget why you came. Some people are greeted with explosions of pleasantries spilling into the present moment while others get garbage bags full of useless memories. But, here you have this pound Puppy, feral Cat, spoiled Horse, or aggressive Iguana, asking: "What the hell is Meg talking about? What storage unit? And what does this have to do with me? Or Flower Essences?" I, Meg, am talking about what could hit you in the head when you open up <u>the emotional storage locker</u> of that animal standing in front of you.

Behavior: Action, reaction, or function under specified circumstances.

The release trigger could be circumstantial, situational, or hit accidentally. When I am being chased out of a corral by a horse as big as an SUV or being growled at by a cat or dog; these are not the times I stop and ask lengthy psycho-babble questions. All these behaviors are noted on the run (sometimes literally) and addressed by choosing appropriate Essences to raise the opposing virtues in this particular personality.

How Do Animals Learn?

Don't have a clue. Sorry. You'll have to ask them. For years, I used to keep up on all the latest tests, results, data, and theories but every time I had one memorized, one of two things would happen. Either new data would replace the old, new data or I would meet an animal who hadn't read that particular scientific study and acted, reacted, or behaved contrary to the published research.

Best advice is to let them tell you WHO they are by HOW they behave.

With that personalized information; you can better solve their unique challenges and problems. Remember, animals (including humans) who have lived under stress or trauma—whether one incident or chronic, long-term—have possibly had portions of their brains eaten away. Stress hormones released in large quantities acting as "brain acid" destroy specific parts of the brain that, for one thing, control impulsive behavior. So it is now, for those animals, a physical limitation. Nonetheless, the majority of these animals who previously had no "PAUSE" in their reactive behaviors, do improve and live purposeful lives using Essences. Even the most desperate cases: give them a chance and see if it is possible to help.

Shorty Growling at his new GrandMother.

All we did was remove his collar. Obviously, he had issues with that. This Pit bull mix, Shorty, had been fostered and shuffled around to 6 fosters in 3 years, verified by vet records from across the state. My son and his wife had Shorty for 2 days and brought him over to meet the rest of the family. I did as I always do and sat far away, made no eye contact, and no sudden movements. Everything appeared to be going fine when Abbey removed his collar and leash. Within a minute, Shorty began to growl with raised hackles and slowly left Abbey's side and moved in my direction. I unfolded from the floor like a Yogini and walked away. Abbey grabbed Shorty and we were safe. But, if he would have been a pouncer; I'd have already been bitten. Or a reactive dog, Abbey would have been bit grabbing him. With weeks of daily Remedies and minimal outside stimulation and little human or canine interaction (he proved to be dog aggressive as well); Shorty got better. He improved so much that he now goes to dog park weekly, gets discounts at doggy day care because he plays so well with other dogs and all caretakers say they love to have him visit. The same dog that 6 other families had relinquished.

Dog Parks, The Urban Phenomena

True story. I took my PERFECT 7 year old, 120 pound German Shepherd to his first fenced dog park. He did great. However, I got into a fight. Absolutely true. A woman brought a hyper Pit bull with no manners and no listening skills to the park where 3 families and 4 dogs had been playing together for a half hour. The Pit bull came in and forced every dog there to roll over on their backs and submit. If they did not as in the case of a large Pointer, the Pit chased him all over the park, knocking down children and pushing adults until the Pointer jumped on a picnic table where his family was sitting. Now the children were crying and the adults were angry.

I stood up and yelled: Get control of that dog.

She yelled back: He's not doing anything wrong.

I yelled: Yes. He is. Get a leash on him.

She yelled: No. He is just doing what dogs doooo.

Within minutes, all the original families had left the park with their dogs and the Pit bull was now alone. When I walked past the owner, she said: "You need to learn about dogs. You, you, you need to watch Animal Planet on TV."

The second time was watching punishment for breed specific behavior.

A young man, mid-twenties, a wife with a baby carriage, and a Husky-Malamute on a harness. I watched as the sled dog loved her pulling, leaping off her front feet to get traction and pull. She loved this and looked beautiful and athletic as she did it. But, every time she did what came naturally as the owner pulled on her harness, she got pulled back harder by the man. Finally, this escalated to him hitting her hard on the top of the head when her front feet left the ground. Yes. Of course, I said something. I have yet to learn that when you reprimand or embarrass; the ignorant perpetrator will often punish more to prove themselves the boss. This is what happened. Regrettably, I left so she would not get hit again…

My bad behavior at Dog Beach.

Reinforcing negative behavior, even for a few minutes, IS DANGEROUS. And if it does not immediately bite you in the ass; the bite may be delivered to someone else's. Case in point is my Border Collie at Dog Beach watching 2 surfers with a Frisbee. It was only a matter of time. Here is what I heard: "I have a dog at home that loves to be teased with a Frisbee. We play 'keep away' all the time. We are here at the beach every day playing with dogs."

I ask: Border Collies?

They answer: Yes. Dogs.

(Raise your hand if you know the difference.)

I knew better. My Border Collie had had enough. She quickly grew tired of their teasing 'Monkey in the Middle' game and started her own game. Higher, faster with more dogged determination to get that Frisbee. Her tenacity is what got the players in the end. No, literally, in the end. One Surfer teased. My Dog leapt. That Surfer threw. My Dog latched. That Surfer was bit. Not his derriere. Just the 5ml of neoprene covering his derriere. She got the Frisbee and won the game. The despots had been warned 10 times not to tease her but my fault for not putting her back on leash. In my pitiful defense, this was "dog" beach; not "surfers in their wetsuits playing Frisbee without their own dogs" beach.

Here is a good story of intervention.

I took my young riding students to a horse show. Very fancy box seats donated to us by a friend. We were right next to the arena watching a jumping class. Everything was going well until one horse kept refusing to jump a large, scary jump. The owner used her whip. The more embarrassed and scared she got; the more she used her whip. My students were horrified because they were never allowed whips, spurs, or any restrictive equipment. This was all happening right in front of our fancy box seats and we were all getting pretty upset. It proved too much for one GrandMother in our group. She stood up tall and in her loudly flowered dress and loudly yelled:

"Hey. Asshole."

(Long pause)

"You hit that horse one more time and I'm gonna come in there and take that whip away from you."

(Very long pause)

Horse and rider looked where the shouting had originated. Both made eye contact with our loud heroine. The whip was lowered and not another blow was struck as the horse and rider left the arena.

Back to improving animal behavior thus, helping humans.

If the change is sudden and drastic without provocation—I go to Star of Bethlehem for shock. This Flower does not care about reviewing a completed questionnaire; it acts. Aconite is good if aggression is involved. This calm, innocuous Flower has power behind its graceful stature and azure colors. Almost like tripping the Giant chasing you. Takes the power away from what you fear.

Hyper-focused animals lack the ability to focus on anything else but the ball, toy, or object of obsession. Your voice, your presence, and your gestures do not exist when neurosis, such as The Frisbee Syndrome, has been activated. Sorry. They can't help themselves. In this case, the opposite virtues are calm focus, multi-tasking abilities, and a new request: LEAVE IT! For these, I'd recommend Impatiens for increased patience; call it a pause button that gets in the way of the next impulsive action. I'd also use Clematis for focus, waking up out of that dreamy state where reality does not exist. Cherry Plum works beautifully for momentary insanity, allowing a nanosecond of relaxation in the situation to recognize that everything is actually OK without succumbing to the obsession at hand. This combination will give you the opportunity to introduce a request like LEAVE IT and the time to get a recognizable response to your request.

"Recognizable response" is a great phrase to mark the behavior. A Labrador chasing a ball, a barking Chihuahua, or a Siamese spraying your couch almost look like they are in a state of euphoria. Right? Eyes dreamily wandering out of focus. Don't even notice your presence until you raise your voice. Their eyes dart back and forth from what they have or want and then back to you, the Spoil Sport. See that moment—when they are able to make a positive choice and listen to you, mark that with a verbal cue like LEAVE IT or a unique sound that will forever mean: LEAVE IT. Make sure either they have already taken the action or immediately follow through. You have to be quicker than they are. Some prefer to clap their hands or use a sound or a gesture like throwing your hands in the air or running to the treats. Next time or two, be careful they are not imitating something without any meaning to them in order to get you to act silly or run and fetch their toys or treats!

Positive, new behaviors should be marked with new words, sounds or signals. If you have been chasing around the Yorkie or Jack Russell during bad behavior yelling: "Don't. Quit. Stop." Get into the game using your Remedies and when you see their "old negative activity" escalating; say: "Uhuh. Shhhht. Enough." Something NEW to mark the soon-to-follow NEW behavior. Next time, when they HESITATE to mark, bark, scratch, or lunge; go crazy with praise. Crazy! Lots of woohoos or attaboys, treats, favorite toy, big loves and hugs. Or leave them alone to chew, relax, or just take a break.

Utilize whatever turns your animal around looking for more of the same positive rewards and recognitions. Within days or weeks using Essences and praiseworthy rewards, this improved behavior will be the more than sufficient reward encouraging more of the same—building on the positive. Let the animals' conscious choices and positive behavior stand alone being the reward in and of itself. Build on that and the sky is the limit.

> One of my greatest personal rewards came when a student got her Thoroughbred gelding to behave perfectly after several failed attempts. We were both in shock because this perfect and brand new behavior was such a stretch for this "bad boy." I yelled: "Reward him. Now." She gathered her reins and galloped right at me. I was pissed because she was losing her window to reward the behavior. As they got closer, I yelled again: "Reward him!" Still running right at me, she yelled: "You are his biggest reward." Awwwww. No really. Awwwww. When they arrived, there were lots of hugs and attaboys.

90% of all aggressive behaviors, in my opinion, stem from fear and/ or confusion. Fear and confusion are littered all over most of these emotional storage units! As well as boatloads of regret, disappointments, and sadness filling to the brim. In some cases, simply looking in their general direction will get you a reaction. Actual eye contact can push a body over the edge. Again, I want to say most of the time, they cannot help themselves as the stress or trauma has "re-set normal" in their lives. Since there is no visible list or inventory of character defects and their triggers; instead, notice negative behaviors as they surface and increase the opposing beneficial quality using the appropriate Remedy.

Situational Rehabilitation—one at a time or by the hundreds as at Katrina; Remedies will be the same and used in the same quantities— several drops per animal no matter their size or weight—and with the same frequency—4-6 times daily. One persnickety kitten on your couch or dozens in a public shelter—same amount and same frequency. Also good news, as mentioned elsewhere, is that Flower Essences work no matter how long ago the personal transgression happened to the animal whether last night's storm or trauma and stress from years ago.

Daisy, the NYC 9-11 dog, is an example. Her loud noise phobia started after she witnessed the Twin Towers come down while home alone. For the next 6 ½ years, every single time there was a loud noise near her Manhattan apartment, she would go to the same window sill and shake uncontrollably... until she got the Flower Essences blended specially for the Katrina animals.

Phobias without known origins

For years, I thought loud noise phobia was a breed specific behavior like Papillions or German Shepherds with big ears. My Shepherd, Tiger, acted anxious when our local Marine base practiced with live artillery. Tiger would pant excessively, climb off and on the couch, walk around the room, want to go out and immediately wanted to come back in. This could go on for hours and (I thought) with no way to comfort him or get him to be still. My friend said: "Use some of your own Remedies." Stupidly, I lectured her on breed specific behaviors. An hour later, at wit's end, I tried some Remedies. Immediately, he settled down. And was sleeping soundly with the artillery still booming. But would it work on the upcoming 4th of July?

At 6:00p.m. on the Fourth of July, I loaded up Tiger's drinking water, put some drops in his dinner, sprayed his chest and then some on my hands and we went to the couch to watch a movie. I forgot about the anticipated nervous behavior. When the revelry started a few hours later with city sponsored fireworks echoing off the hillside and neighbors celebrating with pots and pans, horns honking and the occasional gun exploding; my Shepherd continued to sleep. He slept through it all. Finally, at about 9:00 with this unnatural behavior, I grew worried and woke him up just to make sure he was OK. He got up, stretched with front feet on the ground and rear end still on the couch, got down, had a drink of water, and climbed back up to resume his sleep. NOTHING. Not a thing. No fear, no panting. NOTHING.

"It was like he forgot he was afraid."

Tiger forgot he was afraid of loud noises. After this breakthrough, he never reacted again to thunderstorms, noisy neighbors, or the Marine's live artillery practice. I did more experimenting to prove the efficacy of eliminating phobias. Tiger hated getting his nails trimmed. He showed teeth to the vet. And he liked this vet. We did the same 4th of July Remedy. First time, he was a little better. No teeth showing and a touch less struggling to get free. Second time, no teeth appeared and only pulled back a few times.

A month later, we were getting his nails done, I had the Remedies on Tiger, had a good hold on his 125 pounds, and was ready for the nail trim and said:

OK you can start.

She said: I'm done.

I said: No really. I have a good grip.

She said: No. really. I'm done.

Tiger was over his fear! He never needed Remedies again. The behavior change was permanent after only three applications in three months.

Does not matter if there is one particular defect like only on Tuesday mornings barking when the garbage truck arrives. Or the dog who can't stop barking whether crated, on daily walks, or playing at doggy park. Same goes for multiple personalities like a cat that snarls, growls, claws furniture, sprays, hisses, bites, and hides—all at the same time. Essences can correct all these behaviors by raising the positive qualities of the personality, even if you can't see anything positive; give it a try, you'll be surprised.

Leaving this amazing story in the words of the woman who lived through it:

"My two dogs got picked up and taken by the F-5 tornado in Texas last year. I watched them disappear. Days later, they were found 5-6 miles away. They were alive but badly beaten up and emotionally traumatized. Our house had been completely destroyed except for the staircase I was under in what used to be the closet. One of our horses was also picked up by the tornado, she survived but her foal was later euthanized due to injuries sustained by flying debris. Since then, which is almost a year ago, the horses have become herd bound, not being able to be more than 10 feet away from each other—not even if just across the barn aisle.

The dogs were skittish all the time. If there was a storm approaching, the worst one would go to the very back of her dog house, curling up in a tight ball, staying there for hours. We used the same essences as Noel, the orphaned calf. (Another great story of recovery previously published in Natural Horse Magazine.)

In 2-3 days, a profound change happened in the herd. I noticed they could cope better and were actually spread apart in the field—for the first time in a year. I saw dramatic improvement with the dogs the first day. Recently, a few weeks after starting on essences, a storm came through and one of the dogs did not even react. Winds were so strong, we heard sheet metal being torn off and fly past. Worried about my most traumatized dog; I went to her dog house to check on her. She was not there.

I found her in the living room, asleep on her back, legs splayed open, and snoring. **She was sleeping soundly through her worst nightmare.**"

In The Blink of an Eye

The Process of Change is simply:

1. Identifying the problem.
2. Creating the opportunity to change.
3. Setting up for success.
4. Focusing on intention, not on outcome.
5. Recognizing the change.
6. Enjoying the results.

Just in case, it is not as simple as 1-6, read on.

Swallow, Blink, and Think

What is change? It is miniscule. It is inches and ounces. It is an exhale, a twitch of an ear, a blink, a swallow. These are all signs the brain is working. It is being present enough to see these things. It is being part of the present, the present being either the moment or the gift, being actively a part of the process of change.

Every choice (and every change) has a consequence; the ideal is to make it a positive reward. After choosing and giving a Remedy; change will start to happen. The biggest deal is often getting the human to notice the subtle differences. We are used to big deals, and unless there is drama, flair and a bit of the unnatural; we are not satisfied that ENOUGH has happened. We are in the animals' world, their arena if you will, and should be viewing their world without prejudice. Maybe that is where some difficulties begin, namely: in our perception.

Flower Essence Remedies are so subtle and work so gently that their effects often are overlooked and we credit something else. No matter who or what gets credit, the proof is in the change of the personality, the emotions, and/or their thinking process. Every situation and every animal is unique. Blends can be administered once, the desired result obtained and human and animal are fine thereafter. Usually though, there is a process that takes place during the transformation. The process and its length depend on the individual or the situation.

It is possible your animal gave the best, new behavior behind your back. Possible you missed the TRY and think you have failed to achieve your goal. Careful not to spook the animal into poor behavior. If that happens; apologize and try again.

Special Cases

Rescues and animals in need of rehabilitation suffer from difficulties evident in the added emotional baggage to their lives that as they are made comfortable in their new surroundings and begin to relax and trust, their new companions; ISSUES manifest and begin to create chaos in their new, ordered world. During the process of change, a myriad of behaviors can surface, just recognize and address each one.

<u>Remember to not deplete yourself as you care for others.</u>

Five vets had 5 different opinions but as each of these behaviors manifested, we administered Blends and within the week, the behavior disappeared. After weeks of enjoying the "new" personality, another challenge would arise and the mare had to deal with something else. We addressed each behavior as it arose and she is a beautiful, happy girl now but this process took us months as she revealed more and more to us, using only 3 Blends, one week at a time.

NOTE ON MIRRORS: *This mare was owned by an errant teenage runaway girl. Mom used the same Blend on the teenager after she saw the mare changing. The teenager was rebellious and with no desire to change her "fun" behavior. She refused to actively participate in the training of her mare and wanted no part of Essences. So her Mom would go to her daughter's room at night while the daughter slept and sit with her. The Mom put Essences on her own hands, then gently stroked her sleeping daughter's hair, telling her how much she loved her and that she understood what she was going through, and that things would change for the better. Within 3 weeks, the teenager no longer chose to run away from home. Her grades improved, and so did her relationships within the family.*

Challenges

Use apparent setbacks to your advantage because they could simply be a pop quiz. When the animal is "tested" and holds firm to the new identity, the new way of handling situations, reacting with calm acceptance and knowledge rather than the old way of fight, flight, fright, or freeze; then you have a mark, a touchstone of your progress. Your animal will emerge from each of these testing episodes more convicted and integrated into their new self.

Setbacks can be helpful in convincing us that change has indeed occurred. Challenges will arise and you may think the Essences aren't working. Use these opportunities to gauge where you and your animal exist on the "improvement scale."

A highly accomplished agility dog, after years of competing, decided to not finish the last half of the course no matter what enticements or punishments were offered. His M.O. was to just jump over the small fence after finishing half the course and run away. First time he got these Remedies—Impatiens for patience and Clematis for focus—was at a national competition where the handler had little in the way of expectations that the dog's behavior would be any different here than at her training facility.

Surprise. This dog did complete the first half and then, as expected, jumped over the short fence and ran away. The handler was un-nerved and started to go after him when the dog, on his own, jumped back into the agility ring at the exact same exit spot and finished the course perfectly—without its handler.

A Knock on the Door

Let's say the dog you are working with is reacting to people in the hallway of your apartment building. Could it be that when you hear people talking and laughing and the closer they get to your door, the more tense you become? Maybe, without awareness, you start to "posture" and move toward your dog to grab him/her by the collar and hold them before they can bark. They see you "posturing," ready to pounce and yell. Before you know it, the dog is out of your reach, bolting for the door and barking fiercely at the air. Same applies to asking your animal to get in the car while you nervously hold their vet records in your hand.

Pop Quizzes

Ask yourself:

Does this animal understand what I am asking of him?

Did I miss the try?

Does the animal "see" the result we are requesting? Is that result a reward?

Is there any discomfort, physical pain involved?

Are we asking for the impossible?

Is there any pay-off for your animal NOT doing what you request?

Just because your dog will sit and stay for 30 seconds at your front door does not mean he will do it the first time out at the doggie park. Might have to wait one night, a few days, or even weeks to successfully obtain the new behavior. Be patient and wait for the change. To most, it is as down-to-earth as a tilt of the head, an ear twitch, a swallow, or the blink of an eye.

Test the Teacher

Create a situation in order to mark improvement. Try this. You hear the people in the hall, you reach for a treat, the dog's attention is averted from the hall to you, recognize that moment, treat him/her, give a rub or pat, or a symphony of praises and kind words. And when they don't bark or bolt for the door, treat again. Another way for future fun = when that dog or cat gives you the quickest nod, eye contact, acknowledgement = touch the tip of your nose and then treat. Sometimes you start treating with the hand that is touching your nose. Later treat with the opposite hand so that they will maintain eye contact and not follow the treat. Make sense?

For the horse afraid of or angry at the shoer: practice using appropriate Essences and "play" with your horse with chaps and a hammer, holding the foot longer each time and letting them rest and be comfortable. Find if their anxiety is visual, tactile or auditory and play the game accordingly. With the small animal, "play" getting in and out of the car on days other than scheduled vet visits. Work with your vet to eventually arrive at the office and NOT have an appointment. Maybe just a treat or "atta-boys" when the job of arriving (or being in the exam room) has been met with success.

STICK WITH YOUR INITIAL AGREEMENT

For example, maybe your initial arrangement (part of a training plan) with your animal was to get them safely and quietly to the groomers without an appointment. Walk in and walk out. Say that goes well—DO NOT add "up on the table" near the wash tub, pick up a paw for nail trim. Bring out a power tool. NO. That is out and out lying to your animal. You are breaking your original agreement. Why should they easily trust you again? You can trick them again. Sure. Trust is more important than getting your way.

TRUE STORY: I had a 1,250 pound Clydesdale-Thoroughbred named Bubba that decided he did not like the horse trailer anymore and did not want to leave the farm. Or that he was too in love to go anywhere without his red-headed companion. Whatever his reason—the result was NOT getting in the trailer. He would stand there all day long but not get in. If I got impatient and angry—so did he. If I stood and waited—so did he. But one thing was true—he was not getting in that trailer. So, tricks and treats being exhausted; I decided to tell him the truth.

"We are going to Cloverdale Ranch down the hill."

Nothing.

"We will be back at 3:00."

He walked in the trailer.

No, I am not lying. I have witnesses. We were all so shocked, none of us thought to close the trailer door. That is until he started to walk back out.

I said again: "Three o'clock." He walked right back in. Without exhaling, I closed the trailer door, jumped in the driver's seat, and drove to the ranch. Bubba taught me to tell the truth.

Can't, Didn't and Won't.

No scientific methods exist to prove these Essences are successful because no technology or equipment exists that can measure an Essence. Modern science has nothing to test, prove or disprove the intelligence and gifts of these plants. We can only stand back as did early scientists and use observation as our solitary tool.

Companions who claim no change must ask some serious questions of themselves and their charges:

> Is there a physical ailment or limitation that should be addressed by a health care professional?
>
> Are there any mental deficiencies that prevent the animal from working or thinking at its maximum?
>
> Has the best possible environment been provided?
>
> Was the desired result possible? With this animal? Within this environment?
>
> Was it the appropriate Blend? In the right dosage and frequency?
>
> Was there change but you missed it? Was it not the behavior you were looking for but the one that this animal needed?
>
> Do you need to modify your expectations?
>
> Do you need to see if you are part of the problem?

Since Flower Essences are both subtle and gentle in their effectiveness, it allows some observers to claim that while they do see real change, it is the result of something other than the Essences. People cite time, natural progression, their personal efforts of positive thought or claim there never was any problem.

Flower Essences will work for everyone, notwithstanding severe physical limitations. However, they are not recommended for everyone. Some people prefer to stay "stuck" or if you will—keep the drama, the imbalance or the difficulty in their lives and, consequently, are not honestly looking for resolution.

Phenomena of the Invisible

The phenomenon of seeing these Essences work is not so much that we see the change but is that the human counterpart has the patience to wait, acknowledge, and accept the improvement. Regrettably, sometimes, the Blends don't appear to work because to allow the change in the animal would create a difference in the Companions' life. No blame, just a fact.

Often our animals mirror our needs, be they positive or negative. One friend said since she was not well, it stood to reason that her animal would eventually mirror this condition and compromise his health. Another friend keeps telling everyone her dog is depressed. "Look at her. How sad. Poor thing. She's been like this ever since my boyfriend left us." We all have met at least one person who talked about their jealous cat, their yappy dog, their high strung horse, their finicky eater, etc.

A thought... In the process of getting an animal "right" we have to make sure that we have not become the creator of getting the animal "wrong." Could be we anthropomorphize (give human traits to animals) and destroy the animal's uniqueness. Just a thought.

You Are Not Going to Change 50+ Million Years of Evolution in Your Backyard.

Domestication, with its restrictions and isolation, has created a whole new set of problems for animals they are not emotionally, physically, nor mentally "wired" to deal with. Border collies are designed, not only physically but mentally, to run upwards of 55 miles every single day working their minds and bodies. We bred that into them as working (for humans) dogs. Horses are built—hardwired for 50 million years—to graze and walk 16 hours a day.

Humans have assumed power over domestic animals' freedom, identity, social order, dignity, health, decision-making, and problem-solving capabilities. We put them into stressful situations through training, difficult environments, and restrictions often creating confusion, pain, illness, and then we expect them to behave "appropriately." Restriction can cause build up of pressure, in many cases, resulting in significantly excessive personality traits. We have to contend with or correct what we possibly created.

My Thoughts on Training Cats

Honestly, what else is there to say?

Most of the following stories and case studies were previously published in Natural Horse Magazine and other publications. Thanks to the efforts of wonderful editors—these now follow some rules and order. I have added follow-ups to a few when appropriate. Please don't be prejudice against horses, who occupy the majority of these cases, instead, listen to the importance of the overall message.

Flowers are non-discriminatory and help whoever needs help. That is the reason I tell people, with non-aggressive or severely re-active animals, to put the Essences on their own hands and then gently pet or massage creating a win-win situation. I know we do not intentionally bring our favoritism or our personal drama to the table, but sometimes we can't help ourselves. Please open your hearts and minds to all the animals here and see the similarities, not the differences. Instead, listen to these stories wearing your Cat, Dog, or Elephant ears.

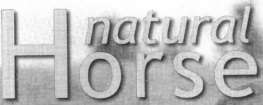

natural
Horse
MAGAZINE   *dedicated to your horse*

HELP THAT SORE BACK with ACUPRESSURE

FOALHOOD: Bring On the FLOWER ESSENCES!

Fight FUNGAL INFECTIONS with CHINESE HERBS and ESSENTIAL OILS

GROUND DRIVING through FEEL

JULY/AUG 2009
Volume 11 Issue 4 $6.95 US

www.naturalhorse.com

CLOUD and the AMERICAN MUSTANG: Secret BLM Plans Revealed ... FINAL DAYS FOR ALL?

Case Studies with Names & Faces

Part One—
Practical Applications for Flowers, Weeds, & Trees

Folklore, Folkmedicine, Folks

Folklore tells us people observed animals choosing certain plants used at time of birthing, injury, or seasonal changes, and people then chose remedies based on what the animals chose. For centuries, herbalists, folk doctors, and caretakers have chosen local plants for the well-being of those in their care. Now it is our turn to choose remedies for our domesticated animals.

When I started using flower essences 40 years ago, the only ones available were from the repertoire of Dr. Edward Bach, British homeopathic physician and discoverer of flower essence therapy. From 1930 to 1936, Bach discovered, researched, demonstrated, documented, and taught others his simple system comprised of 36 plants and trees, one unique source of water (Rock Water essence), and one blend of 5 flowers known as Rescue Remedy. His idea was to keep Flower Essence Therapy in the hands of the layperson, not scientists or other doctors and that is exactly what he did in his research, teachings, and proliferation of his unique discoveries.

Many who study Bach say his work is complete and these are the only agents ever to be used in flower essence therapy. However, I disagree having never read anywhere that Bach declared his research concluded. My thought is, if Dr. Bach had not died at such a young age, he would have given us more than 38 remedies.

Conversely, I do not believe we need thousands of exotic and rare essences as marketed today. I invite you to choose plants based on accessibility and commonality. What I tell people is that animals and humans are not so complicated. Our emotional needs are simple, yet sometimes difficult to provide for in certain settings. Sometimes outside help is needed to smooth personality excesses, bring out hidden potential, or help overcome damage to mind and emotions.

Use an herbalist's mind when choosing a plant or tree to make an essence—try to take into account all aspects of the plant, or at least the glaring ones. For example, consider its appearance, where it has chosen to grow, how, or when. Is it invasive, showy, and demanding attention, like the passion flower? Delicate and wispy like clematis? Does it grow in a place with a far-reaching history (mustard)? Does it grow where it is needed (arnica)? Obnoxiously cheery and bold personality (dandelion)?

Flower Essences

Aconite—Be courageously willing. For personalities prone to sensitivity and restlessness. Never quite focused on the person or task in front of you. Historically Monkshood, Wolfsbane was used for shock, numbness, fear, sensitivity, and sudden fright.

Agrimony—See things as they truly are. Confront and change old negative behavior patterns, living conditions, values. Step into personal, positive authorship of your own life. Transformation for personalities that hide behind an acrimonious face masking their true feelings.

Angel's Trumpet—This highly poisonous plant, when used as a flower essence, helps foster trust and acceptance of change without fear. Recognize the best in any situation. Datura, 15 species worldwide including jimson (loco) weed, is a violently toxic and deadly plant historically used in suicides, thus the nickname, people who used Datura would soon hear the angel's trumpet.

In an essence, this plant allows people to see the best in themselves and in others; it helps with inner conflict, a need for drastic change, adaptation to existing circumstances or else be overwhelmed by them, as in the Gulf region post-Katrina. Some chose to stay and rebuild while others chose to move away and still others chose to succumb—suicides tripled in the Gulf region in the year following Katrina.

Angel's Trumpet was the first to bloom in New Orleans post-Katrina in a neighborhood next to the French Quarter. It was New Year's Day 2006 when we spotted this huge flower in front of an abandoned home with "FEMA Graffiti"—spray painted symbols noting date, searchers' affiliation, number rescued, and number of bodies in the house. Notes about animals were often written on door. The graffiti was a grim reminder of the disaster 4 months previous, but the Angel's Trumpet flowers were a sign of renewal and rejuvenation, moving forward while recognizing and realizing our personal and collective best.

Apple—Cleanse negative self-image. Apple personality is fresh, complicated, bittersweet, impossible to categorize, refreshing, with potential to mature and grow into best version of self. Habitual thought does not make fiction fact.

Arnica—For emotional relief post-trauma. Cleanses hurtful memories. Helps in reconnecting to life after suffering any loss of security such as an accident. Excellent for the overly sensitive personality and for fear of touch as in cases of abuse.

Folklore has it that arnica was first used after people observed mountain goats in the Alps seek out the arnica plant (reportedly eating it and rolling in it) for relief after suffering an accident or injury. Arnica in its natural herbal form is highly toxic to humans and should never be used internally, but in homeopathic form, Arnica Montana enjoys a great reputation among athletes for muscle soreness, bruising, and strain due to overexertion. Those in need of it do not recognize exhaustion and continue on in a state like shock, often to greater injury.

Bleeding Heart—For the worst draining and inconsolable grief. Feeling "bled dry" of your own life force after a loss.

Cherry Plum—For composure and to resist the immediate impulse to mis-behave. For the personality who can't relax in the moment to see that everything is actually OK. Mentally fighting to not behave impulsively and make poor choices. I equate this to a "pause button" on the remote control governing emotions, thinking, and influencing behavior.

Clematis—For the personality that is like these delicate flowers with soft, diffused colors, appearing dreamy and unfocused with no interest in simple, daily tasks. The animals who came to me for help seemed to "come alive" with this flower essence remedy. They get an enthusiasm about their life that had been missing. They want to participate and take ownership in decision making. Most were startled by their own interactive behaviors in the beginning because it was so new to them or long forgotten. Clematis is for those in need of stimulation, enthusiasm, and purposeful living.

Clover—Sweetens any task. Friendship strengthener. Brings out the best. Folklore assigns this prolific spring and summer flower as a blood cleanser and hormone balancer. Use white, pink, red—whatever you have.

Dandelion—Dandelion helps those who are in need of change, requiring courage and the self-confidence of a lion. It is for the personality that is often crabby, never satisfied, in need of eliminating deep-seated, negative habits.

Cheerful Dandelion enjoys a reputation as the "Flower of Survival" either because it is among the first to bloom after winter or because it springs back after being stepped on. It is colorful, abundant, and hardy. Historically used as tea, wine, food, and in folk medicine as a "springtime" tonic for eliminating sluggishness. One of my absolute favorites.

Impatiens—Increase patience. Overcome irritability and restlessness.

Impatiens is often overlooked because it is so unpretentious and adaptable and not much is written about this Himalayan flower. It is simple in its elegance and delicacy, yet powerful enough to change a personality. As an essence, Impatiens is one that can never be over-used as most people and animals could do with more patience. Those in need of this essence are impulsive, stubborn, too independent, and/ or confrontational.

Mimulus—Ideal essence for the personality struggling with known fears, lacking conviction and belief in themselves to overcome a challenge.

This flower is actually shy, delicate, sensitive and found in extremely harsh environments. Sometimes a plant makes a statement as to what it can accomplish, as in the case of Mimulus being a delicate flower nonetheless growing in the most adverse conditions. It blooms only for several weeks and disappears if conditions become unfriendly or too harsh. If circumstances are not beneficial, Mimulus can lay dormant, hiding for years.

Mustard—Despair is the word most often used by Dr. Bach in describing the Mustard personality which suffers from lingering depression.

Excellent example of where a plant chooses to grow and flourish, which is usually exactly where it is most needed. The Mustard I gather is found growing prolifically in front of the San Luis Rey Mission in California. This marks the spot where many years ago, hundreds of Native American families were torn apart and the strong ones were forced to work within the walled confines of the Mission. They were forbidden to speak their native languages and practice their ceremonies, required to cut their hair, wear shoes, submit to physical punishment. Mustard grows spectacularly at this exact spot where the families were first separated and later would secretly meet, only to have to part again before getting caught.

Oak—Endurance, driven by sense of duty, fighting against rest until exhausted, describes the Oak personality.

"My" oak tree is a live coastal oak at 6,000 feet atop Palomar Mountain in San Diego County, California. This oak is upwards of 400 years old. If magic were ever going to be used to describe a tree or a forested area, this is the time and place. During the summer, when the tree was at its zenith, I placed some oak leaves in a glass bowl of water and let it potentize all night during a total lunar eclipse, during the following day in the sunshine, and again that night in the actual full moon. We call it: Oak Moon-lite Essence.

Passion Flower—Comfortable correction. Good for the personality that is aggressively making mistakes and needs gentle guidance to improve itself and its behavior.

Flourishing, gorgeous, multi-faceted flowers with tendrils that have apparent kinetic energy to reach for objects, elegantly attach itself, and climb. We once had a very cranky neighbor. He was antagonistic claiming a boundary dispute and said he was going to "exercise his rights as a property owner" utilizing an easement he marked off without benefit of a survey. I did not have the means nor the energy to fight him and instead planted Passion Flower along the disputed fence line. The flowering vine grew and flourished. Months later, official documents surfaced, revealing he and his fence actually encroached 20 feet onto our property (along the entire length of 900 foot fence). He was forced to correct his mistake.

Pine—Grow strong where you are planted. Draw on others for strength and good orderly direction.

Rock Rose—Overcome sudden shock. Restore hope. Remain steadfast. (One of my personal mainstays.)

Rose—Positive self-sufficiency.

Take a close look at the entire picture or process. Great for birthing as well as all transitions. Not like 'rites of passage' Agrimony. More like the sophisticated and elegant answer to life's changes and challenges. Being wise not clever. Being calm not detached. Having integrity, understanding, and reliability.

Rosemary—Feel safe and secure in your choices on your personal path.

Like un-covering there always has been and always will be a divining force guiding your choices; intuition that never lets you down. FEELING LUCKY 24/7/365. To safely and easily seek your own answers—being loyal to yourself. Increases inspiration, self-esteem, and loyalty. Said to be a gift from the Greek Goddess, Aphrodite and also the Roman Goddess, Venus. Broad spectrum of practical and ceremonial uses in many varied forms. Named "rose of the sea" because historically sailors could smell Rosemary long before they could see land giving them feelings of comfort, security, and safety—without any doubt, knowing they were on the right course.

Star of Bethlehem—For shock or trauma of any description.

Star of Bethlehem is rumored to have been Dr. Bach's favorite flower essence for treating shock. This is the only single remedy (all others were Flower Essence blends) I brought to the gulf region in September 2005, which proved itself indispensable. I dealt with hellacious post-Katrina situations as short-term manager of a barn full of critical care veterinary patients, all the cats, all the birds, all the exotics, snakes, and 150 aggressive dogs evacuated to Gonzales, LA. There were nearly 400 animals in this barn on any given day and 2,000 on premises.

After seeing how I was using Star of Bethlehem and making decisions quickly and confidently, a volunteer asked for my last bottle when headed to the hospital with a life-threatening spider bite. He and his family were shocked by the severity of the bite and uncertain of what the future held. He returned the next day after 2 emergency surgeries with a good prognosis. The family had drained the bottle!

Sweet Pea—For round-the-clock kindness.

Sweetgrass—Offers a deep feeling of security. Appreciate and welcome change. Ease tension in the moment.

I "discovered" Sweetgrass flower essence when long blades of Sweetgrass, sent from an Iroquois family in Canada, were soaking in a bowl of water to soften in order to braid and then dry for burning in a Native American ceremony. As soon as I saw the water, I said: "I'll be having that for an essence." My family and friends are always my first proving grounds. After each of us had a sip of the fresh Sweetgrass water, we fell asleep on each other like a litter of puppies. We slept soundly with contentment and comfort. This was during the summer of 2005 and within 2 months, introduced it in a blend for Hurricane Katrina victims to provide a feeling of security and reassurance.

Tiger Lilly—Promotes companionship and sense of team spirit.

For the companion lacking in thoughtfulness and consideration necessary in any give-and-take relationship. Bring out hidden gifts and potential like the dots "hiding" inside the petals of this Lily. Foster the sense of being part of something greater than yourself—not egotistical but more in an attitude of self-sufficiency while your individual contributions make the team stronger.

Yarrow—Thrive and flourish in hostile environments.

Clarify personal boundaries in any group setting. Rise above your present circumstances or surroundings when the situation itself can't be improved—shelters, zoos, schools, work places, natural disasters, intimidating or overwhelming negativity of any kind.

Excellent for those who are continually asked to accept unacceptable treatment, behaviors, or environments. Draw on mental, emotional resources previously hidden, unused, not yet discovered. Also good for sudden change in environment and violent acts. To some, may be as innocent as crating, carrying, transporting, and depositing at a new location.

Yarrow *Achilles millefolium* is an intriguing plant with a good amount of written folklore. Legend has it a Centaur taught Achilles and his soldiers to stuff Yarrow leaves into arrow and spear wounds to stop the bleeding. The Dakota named Yarrow "medicine for the wounded." For the Wounded Warrior/Hero in order to not to be drawn into negativity of present circumstances and to not be drained—"bled dry" by others or existing negative conditions.

Blending

Blends are like a companion garden, a team, a circle of friends—designed to bring out the singular and collective best in all. The idea is that each unto itself is whole and perfect but becomes a better version of itself when associated with others.

Addiction, abuse, sadness, and recovery all boil down to better choices—easy to say if you are already eating the green, green grass on the other side of THAT fence. Not afraid to speak my PIECE of a solution… in a place where massive amounts of anti-depressants and laxatives are consumed… in our sad, constipated nation.

I do not expect nor want anyone to take my word for IT—IT being the potential of a straightforward solution to help others that is "hiding" inside the plant, flower, stem, leaf, acorn, needle, seed or what have you—begging for acknowledgement. Create your own adventure, your own relationship with the flower, tree or weed that calls to you. There are no secrets in Nature, just answers we may be too impatient to notice or too distracted to accept. Essences of Impatiens and Clematis can help with those limitations.

The Future

Essences are inexpensive, accessible, easy to make, and nothing is harmed during preparation. Dried flowers and plants have been successfully used to make essences, and this may be needed in the near future, considering that some of these plants, trees, and flowers are being wild-crafted out of existence or are endangered from climate change, bug infestation, genetic modification, etc. Dr. Bach probably never imagined a world of changing climate, extinctions, undernourished soil, and contaminated water. But we are there and need to make adjustments, personally and globally.

Not Too Proud to Beg

Bullying, victims, addiction, sadness, mental disorders, and "feelings of being different" plague our nation. I am saying the truth as I see it today—we are in a world where our children are dying from the effects of cruelty every single day. In a room of twenty 10 year olds, 3 have thought IN DETAIL how to kill themselves.

One positive action we can take immediately is try this blend treating children, families, friends, caregivers, and educators alike: Aconite for restlessness and sensitivity, Agrimony for those feeling they are caught in the middle, Angel's Trumpet for confident outlook, Apple for cleansing negative self-image, Clematis for focus and follow-thru, Impatiens for patience, composure, tolerance, Mustard to reduce lingering depression, Rose for positive self-sufficiency, Sweetgrass for welcoming change and encouraging dialogue, Yarrow for surviving, thriving in negative environments. What do you have to lose? Everything.

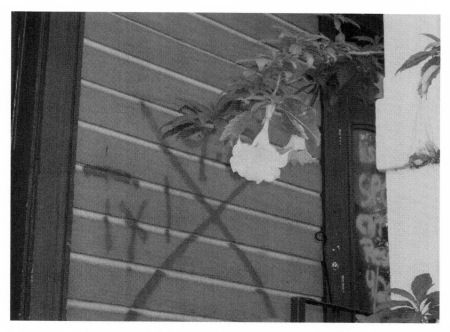

New Orleans Angel's Trumpet and Katrina Graffiti on New Year's Day 2006

As a flower, historically, the highly poisonous Angel's Trumpet is used for assisted suicide—thus the name. Suicides tripled in the Gulf region the year following hurricanes Katrina and Rita. As a Flower Essence, Angel's Trumpet is used to KNOW YOUR BEST and recognizing what you are truly made of… which is always better than you ever thought.

Passion Flower planted for a very cranky neighbor.

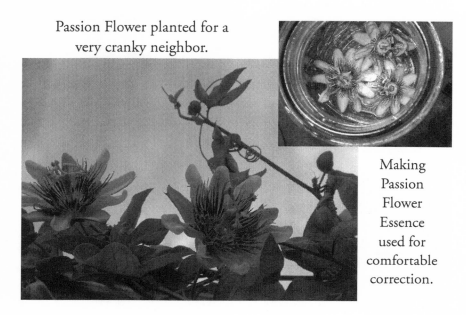

Making Passion Flower Essence used for comfortable correction.

Mimulus flourishing in spite of its difficult environment.

Mimulus Essence is for surviving and thriving in harsh conditions. Overcoming the effects of abuse, neglect, cruelty, and disappointment.

Emotional Safeguards When Home Alone

A night out, a day at the office, or a long vacation are probably all the same difference to our animals left behind. Interviewing professionals and "animal parents" has revealed to me something surprising: worries about animals are identical whether from the parents or the temporary caregivers. These concerns are a change in eating habits and routine, the possibility of separation anxiety, and fear of an illness or accident.

Leaving your dogs, cats, or horses at home with a caregiver or taking them to a boarding facility is a personal choice. Public facilities usually require proof of vaccinations and a certificate of health from a veterinarian. This alone will force many animal parents preferring traditional and natural health care to look for alternatives. If you do choose a facility, check its references thoroughly and visit more than once, especially at feeding times when stress levels can be high. See how the staff handles this routine and see if you feel comfortable with their practices. Either choice will bring up issues to be addressed before you leave so problems can be avoided while you are away. Remedies are identical either for in-home or boarding situations.

Routines

Flower Essence Therapy is highly effective in eliminating and preventing negative behaviors, attitudes, and emotions when routine is broken.

The owners of Pancho, the Chihuahua, left at 4:00 in the morning for Cuba and I arrived at 6:00. Pancho and I had met twice before and got along well, but this morning without benefit of his parents' presence, he decided to bark incessantly and evade my advances to put his leash on for a walk. His "brother and sister" patiently waited for us. Persian rugs and my reputation were at stake. A full slice of his favorite meat with several drops of Chestnut Bud, Yarrow and Sweetgrass flower essences got the leash on without further fuss in less than 5 minutes. The afternoon walk was not a problem using the same remedies as a precaution. He accepted and trusted me after that first day and we all stayed on schedule.

Chestnut Bud flower essence helps break down a complicated process into bite-size pieces, easier for mental digestion. Yarrow is for environment. Even though his actual surroundings had not changed, my presence changed the contents. I have discovered that Yarrow works well for reactive animals. Sweetgrass essence helped Pancho to accept the change of leadership.

Separation Anxiety

Symptoms of this problem are varied but the remedy is simple. Symptoms include aggression and depression and lots of in-between behaviors. Cats hide under the bed or may stop using the kitty litter box. Dogs become toy aggressive. One pet sitter in Florida said a dog growled at him when he went to sit on "her" couch. This reactive behavior of guarding territory can also be a sign of separation anxiety. Use your essences; spray the area. Essences do not need to be ingested to be effective. Wait a few minutes and let the essences do their job. Use every 10 minutes until behavior improves or they cease guarding. New behaviors could also include whining inconsolably, barking incessantly, or yowling in the middle of the night. All of these behaviors can be remedied with flower essence of Dandelion, to help with the re-adjustment of their internal clock.

Quick reference chart of behaviors and flower essences to remedy them:
For Drama Queens = Chamomile
For Anger = Rose
Nervous agitation = Aspen or Sage

Anxiety and worry = Sweetgrass or Gorse
Acceptance of strangers = Passion Flower
Abandonment issues = Dandelion or Sweet Pea
Depression = Mustard or Honeysuckle

Sudden Trauma

Alleviate worry about accidents or illness with a stocked and ready "emotional first aid kit". This kit should include a remedy for sudden illness, accident, or emergency. Star of Bethlehem essence is my favorite and if you only want or can afford one—this is the one. If you think it looks like someone is getting sick or you think there is stress, use this flower immediately. If there is bad weather coming or a big change in environment, use Star of Bethlehem. If there is illness manifested already and the shock has not worn off, use this remedy. It has never disappointed me. Animals respond beautifully to it, as is evident in their calm composure and acceptance of difficult surroundings or circumstances. Aconite essence is also excellent for avoiding taking on the stress and resignation that often accompanies bad news or ill feelings.

Remember some of these remedies are as close as your kitchen or yard. Place (non-toxic) fresh or dried flowers or leaves in good water in glass, place in sun for 20-60 minutes, strain and serve! Refrigerate up to 3 days.

Experts across the board also agree on a few simple tasks that greatly help calm the animals while away:

- Leave on the radio or TV.
- Let the easily stressed ones have a piece of your recently worn clothing to lie with while you are away.
- Don't make a big deal when leaving. *Tell them where you are going and when you will be back.* Tell them the truth. Keep your promise. Don't believe me? Try it first before you doubt it works. And enjoy your time away!

Solutions for the Neglected and Abandoned

Words have great power to influence thinking and action—words like neglect, abandonment, and abuse. Neglect is a word with a history to me because I have been accused of that deed more than once. Let me explain and tell you how I came out the other side.

Twenty years ago I was formidably chastised by my veterinarian and accused of 'neglect' when I refused to no longer vaccinate my adult horses. I was told my horses were going to be the sole cause of an outbreak of influenza and encephalitis and I endangered the health and lives of every horse within a wide parameter of my house. All I could think to say at the time was: "Then you'll probably want to stop petting my dog."

A similar scolding was sent my way when the same vet was informed that I no longer fed a strict Alfalfa hay diet. My neighbors were horrified when I neglected to blanket my horses in the winter: ponies, Quarter Horses, and warmbloods alike. We live in southern California! And there were severe warnings when I neglected to put shoes on my ponies.

This might be a word game to some, but my 2 decades of neglect—reducing my interference into the balanced lives and perfect health of all animals in my care—resulted in no influenza, no encephalitis, no strangles, no colic, no food related illnesses, and no hoof problems. I had to go against 35 years of instruction and habit to accomplish that feat.

PUPPY MILLS

A clear case of neglect and abandonment can be seen in a Louisiana court-ordered seizure of 17 Beagles raised to become hunting dogs. All were individually housed in rabbit cages—small cages without solid flooring, only wire, so feces and urine would not sit in the bottom. There was no daily care, limited exercise, and no human contact for their entire lives.

Peanut, 8 months old, from the LA seizure, became more fearful and confused as kennel workers tried to get him out of his kennel for exercise and socialization. Within a few weeks, Peanut's fear of people grew into aggression and he bit the hands that were trying to get a leash on him. He had to be "poled" (a loop on the end of a 6' pole) to be removed from his kennel and walked with the rigid pole between him and his handler. His appetite started to suffer and his health was at risk.

Lack of socialization with siblings and others in early life is the culprit here. "Puppy mill" animals exhibit a behavior commonly called insecure dominance (interestingly, the same behavior I see often in horses who were imprinted at birth … but that is fodder for another article entirely). Insecure dominant behavior manifests in over-the-top play activities, an attitude at mealtime that is not quite food aggression, or a lack of respect and manners while interacting.

Peanut was placed on the euthanasia list as kennel life was making his aggression worse. Instead, with a miraculous intervention and promises of "no blame", he was brought into our home. He stayed under the bed one whole day refusing all treats and soft words trying to cajole him.

Finally, I sprayed a flower essence blend under the bed—Sweet Pea for the gentle personality victimized by others, Mustard for lingering depression, and Gorse for loss of hope when circumstances appear insurmountable. Peanut was not comfortable on the "outside" and loved living in his "cave" (crate) with his toys, blankets, and essences. We continued with this remedy for 10 days in water, food, treats, and spraying his bedding. By then he then felt comfortable on the outside. When he was ready, we began some training, with the help of additional essences.

Some momentary lapses in positive behavior did occur but overall there was steady progress. Flower Essence blends and a happy home life had Peanut comfortably walking on leash within only 3 weeks of his arrival. He was adopted by a foster family that understood his history, behaviors, and emotional needs. Years later, I heard Peanut was alive, well, and living still with his original foster family in Baton Rouge, Louisiana. The original owner lost his court case and never regained possession of any of his Beagles.

FERAL CATS

Feral means "returned to an untamed state from domestication", usually after being cast out or abandoned. Abandonment is a physical act, but to the animals it is a feeling. That feeling is an emotion, which is typically exhibited in 'negative' behavior. Some act out aggressively, like Peanut. Some shut down and become withdrawn or depressed.

The first cat is abandoned on the streets or in the woods and reverts to wild instincts in order to survive. Offspring are born wild. And on goes that story. I will not enter into debate on what to do about the massive numbers of feral and wild cats in the United States, but I will tell you what to do for those who are captured, whether they are to be released or to become domestic.

Flower essences used for the ferals—the epitome of abandonment—are the same we used post-Katrina for the animals left behind in the flood waters of New Orleans: essences of Sweetgrass for welcoming change, Arnica for loss of security and erasing negative, hurtful memories, and Yarrow for the "wounded warrior".

HE ONLY THOUGHT HE WAS ABANDONED!

Have you slipped quietly out the front door? Or sneaked out the back door? Oh yes you have! Leaving poor Rover at home while you work a second job to pay for his vet, groomer, toys, food, and new furniture destroyed by Rover, the abandoned dog… Use the same flower essences listed above with dogs and cats exhibiting this behavior of separation anxiety.

For the cat left behind, who develops an unhealthy attitude choosing to leave you 'presents' outside the litter box, on your bed, or even in your shoe, consider Passion Flower flower essence. It works wonders for cats leaving you unwanted house gifts. I nicknamed this essence "comfortable correction".

MUSTANGS

Trauma of our American wild horses—being rounded up, possibly separated from family, disposed of in corrals, fed on a schedule with unfamiliar food and water—means *upset on every level*. Many shut down mentally, emotionally, and physically, as also witnessed when domestics meet with trauma that uproots them from anything familiar, such as in the case of natural disasters requiring evacuation.

The following flower essences have been successfully used on wild horses, Katrina victims, and domestic horses, dogs, and cats rescued after having been abandoned for a week in a 2003 California firestorm: Yarrow for environment, Arnica essence and homeopathic 30x to release negative muscle memory stored in the system, Star Tulip for grounding, Star of Bethlehem essence and homeopathic Aconitum 30x for shock, and Clematis for improving mental outlook. One rescue operation had 400-gallon water troughs and needed only one ounce of blends per trough to treat everyone for a week.

"After 5 days and 3 evacuations barely ahead of the fires, my Thoroughbred mare was the only one at (coastal evacuation center) Del Mar Race Track eating, drinking, and breathing normally, only because I used my bottle of remedies intended for fear that we had for shoeing." Rebecca McNulty of Carlsbad, California in October 2003 was in a different part of San Diego County and able to attend to her young horse. Others were forced to evacuate without their animals because the late night fire was fueled by 70mph Santa Ana winds. Several people perished—one woman in Valley Center, California along with her 2 horses, in their trailer that went off the road due to smoke impairing visibility.

Time does not matter when it comes to flower essences' efficacy. What I mean by that statement is that it does not matter whether the transgression or trauma or shock happened years prior or a moment ago. Flower essences, if chosen well, eliminate the cause of the disturbance, be it fear, confusion, shock or anything else. I have not found a behavioral problem that does not respond to essences. In my practice, 1 out of 200 treated will not respond—but that is definitely due to an organic reason and not the limitation of the essence. Another comforting thought is we do not need a complete history of the individual to resolve the negative behavior with flower essences. Therefore they can always be successful on feral cats, abandoned dogs, and wild horses.

With 38 years experience, my personal preference is blended flower essence remedies to address all the facets of less-than-desirable behaviors. Blending essences assures permanent solutions to even the most chronic problems, with a future of the best possible behavior, best thinking and best decision-making possible.

Getting Along with Others, Apologies for All Species

"Why can't everyone settle down and just get along with each other?" An age old dilemma with a simple remedy: Give everyone what they need. Soothe their fears, help them accept change, and help them feel safe in a new environment. How? With flower essences. Flower essences offer immediate resolution to emotional and mental problems faced by animals in any dynamic situation.

Dis-honesty Pays Off

"What are you doing petting that cat? No one has ever gotten close to her. She had kittens and they were all as wild as her."

I had not been 100% honest with this client. I never told her my rapid progress with her young Thoroughbred colts was more due to the flower essences I put on my hands, brushes and tack than to the "whispering" she thought I was doing. Her horses were destined for the track and she liked to keep them a touch on the wild side before sending them out for training. Tremendous progress was possible with these yearlings after using a blend of Angel's Trumpet for trust, Cherry Plum for self-control, Impatiens for patience, Rock Rose for courage and Star of Bethlehem for inner-peace.

This blend meets the individual's needs of trust, bonding, and establishing a give-and-take relationship—requirements to be companions with humans. Obviously, these essences also met the barn cat's needs allowing her to buddy up for the first time with a human. Within days, she also buddied up to the dogs, much to their annoyance.

Wild Dogs

Emotional needs of an animal are not complicated, as observations on 2 wild dogs housed together at an animal sanctuary show … before and after using flower essences. This is what the caregiver recently wrote about the improved behavior:

"Initially, we saw the baring of teeth, stiffness in crossing paths, and total avoidance of each other. Since using the blend created for courage for only a few days, I've seen them lying near one another, play bowing, and I've sensed a much more relaxed atmosphere between the two of them. One used to dart past me and now calmly trots by. The other one is more interested in sniffing me and the area I was just in after I leave. Both have much better appetites, even when we sit with them!"

Consider a combination of Angel's Trumpet essence for trust and "knowing your personal best", Mimulus for known fears, double doses of Rock Rose for steadfastness and courage, Star of Bethlehem for shock, and Star Tulip for grounding and feelings of safety in any existing environment. Sweetgrass is also excellent for welcoming change.

Flowers that Apologize

Bringing home someone new can be catastrophic. If any of your existing family takes the transgression personally and is unable to "get over it", apologize immediately. Perfect flower essences for this are Gentian for the fright (emotional hurt) to the heart, Mimulus or any of the Monkeyflowers for fear, Arnica for re-alignment of your status in the world, and/or Lady Slipper for grounding. Homeopathic Chamomila 6x is good for older animals accepting unruly youngsters into the fold. For fighting and overt behaviors, use Star of Bethlehem if you have it on hand.

Seeing the positive results of using essences, most people want to expand their repertoire of essences. But often budgets don't allow for dozens of single remedies or blends. So when I am asked "What is the best essence to use?", my answer is: "The one that is in your hand." Trust the world of essences and use the remedy available. I also believe, after 38 years of watching essences work, that plants and animals are not as complicated and as difficult as some think. Animals are easy to help, simple in their acceptance of our assistance. They can feel our intention to help just as they can feel fear, anger, and distrust.

Remedies for All Species

My first jaunt outside the world of horses, dogs, and cats was with Dude, the iguana. Dude lived in a pet store and had become dangerously aggressive due to rough handling from fearful and inexperienced employees. Because of his behavior, Dude was unadoptable and restricted to living in a wire cage and rarely touched for 4 months when I met him. The employees, unfamiliar with flower essences, challenged me to help Dude. There was one young girl willing to pet Dude through the wire.

I used the same essences proven to restore abused horses and dogs that have turned aggressive. I put several drops, on the girl's right hand, of Gorse for hope, Mimulus for fear, and Gentian for hurt feelings. Then she touched Dude with her left hand, not putting any of the remedy directly on him. Immediately, Dude rolled his eyes up, and his skin softened and was easily rotated by the caregiver's fingers. The iguana leaned closer to her with his body relaxing against the cage. One young, tattooed and pierced, employee, said: "I'm outta here. This is too spooky for me!"

Three weeks later I went back to check on Dude. He was not in his cage. When I asked where he was, someone told me that his behavior improved so much that he got adopted out to a family. I asked what happened to the bottle of essences and was told they gave the rest of the bottle to a woman with an angry duck!

Because I am a trainer by nature, it is the human-animal bond I work to establish, but essences are effective for all introductions of animals to each other or to new, different species. My experience and research is limited to 15 species (human beings are #15). Feedback has been positive and behavior improvement successful on wild dogs, feral cats, pushy pigs, spooky horses, depressed ferrets, self-destructive birds, stressed chickens, goats, sheep, aggressive pet rats, fearful rabbits, iguanas and angry ducks!

Part Two—Basics and Beyond

Can't Train Trauma

After years of working with rescued and "damaged" horses headed to their end because of bad behavior, I came to believe these horses were, to varying degrees, in a state of shock. Many were so surprised by their inhumane and confusing treatment that they either shut down or became enraged, making them unpredictable and dangerous.

Thanks to flower essences, various dramatic behavior improvements took place that seemed impossible, given the history of the animal or the circumstances. Circumstances included hurricanes, weeklong firestorms, tornadoes and court ordered animal seizures.

Flower essences address current the crises and, equally as important, the past—replacing old, negative memories with healthy, positive thoughts. Effects on the animals' future behavior include giving them the opportunity to learn, and to accept, co-operate with, and trust human intervention and companionship.

Starr

Starr was a horse who taught me the true power of flower essences. This mare arrived at my farm filthy, angry, tense, restless and hating to be touched. I had 30 days to "fix" this horse without knowing how traumatized she was. The owner simply said: "We leave the halter on." He bragged that this gorgeous mare cost only $100 at the monthly auction. He failed to mention that this ½ ton horse had hospitalized 2 people since then.

After he left that first day, I went to take the halter off and saw that the 2-inch buckle was rusted shut. Then I saw the deformed, indented bone on her nose. Her facial bones, as she grew, could not grow where the non-giving nylon yearling halter was, so there were deep indentations in the bones and muscles of her head. How she could have chewed and eaten, I don't know. The cheekbone near the eye was deformed as well, and her poll bones and muscle were indented. Imagine a yearling halter on a grown horse's face… There were many misshapen bones. This halter had been on for years and the bone and flesh grew to fit the halter. I had a choice as to how to proceed and I chose flower essences. No outside help, no surgery, and no more trauma.

To start, flower essences were added to her water, her hay and sprinkled in her new corral: Rock Rose for steadfastness and follow-through, Clematis for learning and focus, Cherry Plum for composure, Impatiens for patience, double doses of Star of Bethlehem for shock and restoration, and Star Tulip for renewed grounding and comfort.

After 3 days of essences, she trusted me enough to cut the halter off her face. The halter hung upside down, the noseband wedged within the bone it shaped, for a full 10 minutes before she moved enough for it to fall out. When she freed herself, I left it there on the ground for the next few days. She urinated on it, struck at it, flung it in the air and urinated on it some more.

During Week 2 I added Crab Apple for improving self-image, Red Clover for control, and Sweet Pea for grounding, to some bath water. She still had a hard time being touched or with fast movements, so she got sponge baths with these essences. I also made a bucket of essences to dip my hands in for light massage and stretches. I had to ease her into moving parts of her body that were stoved up from years of tension.

During Week 3, the essences Gentian for courage and optimism and Mustard for lingering depression were added to her water and feed. The vet said she could never be ridden due to an old injury to the shoulder, probably from a trailering incident. The farrier trimmed her, and even though she cooperated, he doubted she had ever been trimmed, and there was permanent damage as a result of improper feed and exercise.

Armed with this information, we intensified the massages, gave her hydrotherapy, added carrot stretches to the routine, started teaching her tricks to help her become more supple, and put flower essences on her treats. She learned to bow, follow her tail in tight circles, reach back onto her rump to get a treat, paw the air, and to bob and weave.

When it was time for her to go home, her family was taught her tricks in order to keep her supple and comfortable. They also got a 90-day supply of Mimulus for known fears, Gorse for hope, and Impatiens for patience with the humans.

Hurricane Katrina

Hurricane Katrina created tens of thousands of animal victims who needed something special to deal with the trauma of repeated disappointments, abandonment, confusion, and the sense of hopelessness these conditions presented. They needed to overcome the assault of mental and emotional trauma. They needed to accept help from strangers. They needed to accept that some of their families were gone forever.

Thanks to friends and family who believed flower essences would help the Gulf Region animals, we were able to give away 200 bottles of blends to rescue workers and victims. When I first arrived at Lamar-Dixon in Gonzales, Louisiana, which was home to more than 11,000 animals in a 7-week period, the skeptics were afraid I was going to hurt the animals by adding essences to the drinking water. But within 90 minutes, someone yelled: "Bring flowers, we have a stressed out dog over here."

Essences blended together for the dogs, cats, horses, and other Katrina victims were Gorse for hope, Yarrow which is the "wounded hero remedy", Echinacea to balance all subtle systems, Iroquois Sweetgrass for welcoming change, Arnica for loss of security, reconnection, and cleansing hurtful memories, plus 12,000 GrandFathers (stones gathered at 12,000 feet from a glacier in North America) allowing vision and acceptance of the future—that all things will make sense in time. Homeopathics of Aconitum 30x were added for shock, worry, and fear of the future, and Arnica 30x for relief from trauma, stress, and overexertion.

When Hurricane Rita struck later that week, essences were put in all the waters and sprayed throughout the barn. We had the quietest, calmest barn full of 250 rescued dogs, and 5 volunteers asleep on FEMA cots. Yes, we slept through a hurricane.

Months later, some dogs and cats were still not rescued, living under abandoned houses, drinking contaminated water and eating whatever they could find. Deb Rykoff, DVM from Barrington, Illinois and 25-year veteran volunteer with Best Friends Sanctuary said: "We not only used your sprays (above listed formula) in the field rescuing animals, we used them in the trucks transporting, and at staff meetings at the end of a long day."

3 Years Later

I saw Starr's family and asked how she was doing. They said she was wonderful. Even though she was never ridden; she entertained with her tricks at every family BBQ. They also said she was helpful during a wild fire demanding a mandatory evacuation. The family stopped and picked up neighbors' horses, some never trailered before, while Starr kept all of them calm.

Intention of Touch

As you read, think Dog, Pig, Rabbit, Pet Rat, Goat, Sheep, and Bovine personalities because all will benefit.

There is a children's game using only one finger and one refrain: "I'm not touching you." It is a game played until the anxiety and expectation is too much to handle and someone pulls away or gets swatted. Few people are immune to this teasing, even without the words.

Horses play this game reacting to a hovering fly. A muscle twitch, a swish of their tails, or stomping their feet reacting to this "intention to touch." How many times does Alpha Mare have to actually touch another horse to get them to do as she bids? Usually all she has to do is look in their direction to communicate her desires. I try to keep this in mind when approaching a horse to touch, handle, groom, and affix equipment, let alone ride them.

Personalities.

Nervous? Stoic? Flighty? Withdrawn or a bit forward? If they are forward and in your space; they may be telling you a need to protect their space or create an area they can back into if necessary. I don't always find the "forward" horse to be pushy. I am not talking about the bully with his chest puffed up like a rooster or sneaking up breathing down your neck. This article is going to take everything down a notch from how I usually discuss behaviors. Previous articles deal with extreme situations and difficult personalities. Here, I want to talk about subtle cues our more sensitive horses send that may go unnoticed but are shouting volumes of important information.

Added bonus is once we have learned this information from the hypersensitive; we can be more sensitive in our approach to the next one and maybe help to bring them down a notch on their stress or anxiety ladder.

Methods of discovery

15 minutes of observation will tell you lots about the personality you are about to ride, massage, groom, trim, or help in some way. First, take a full minute to check in with yourself. Make sure you are not bringing emotional baggage into the session. Introduce yourself and ask permission to be there, revealing your intentions. Does not have to be out loud, the fly never says anything and its intention is well felt. My personality is to be chatty and when I am quiet; makes me more attentive and in sync with the horse and their immediate needs.

How do you "feel" in front of this half-ton EMOTIONAL STORAGE UNIT? What in the heck is stored inside? Fear, loathing, grief? Love, compassion, trust? And how is it affecting the overall well-being of this particular individual? What else can you learn by just standing there? How do you feel? Is your head swimming with worry? Do you want to shift your weight back and forth from one foot to the other? Are you starting to get nervous? I was taught if I got nervous to "lower everything" including voice, head, blood pressure, and if riding; lower my hands, heels and heart rate.

Experiment.

After you have gathered some information about the emotional and possibly the mental state of this horse; approach any part of the body, hopefully, being offered to you to touch. (Keep in mind that offering you his rear-end is not always a bad thing.) Hover your hand 1-12 inches above the body and while moving slowly—one inch per second to start—see how your horse feels about this. Take inventory. Is he getting nervous? Moving away? Moving into you? Is the breathing changing? Head rising? Eyes more alert? Moving his lips? Moving his feet? Should you back off a bit or is he inviting you in closer?

Check in every few minutes and see how he "feels" and how do you "feel" now? Adjust your non-touching pressure accordingly or maybe take a short break. Some will stay with you wanting more or they could just have good manners and stay close. Maybe they just need a drink. If they walk off; many will walk back to you if you wait. You be the judge how and when to proceed.

Plants have personalities too.

Personality is used here to describe traits and characteristics studied in varied disciplines under names including: doctrines of correspondents and of signatures, laws of similars, contraries and cures. For today's discussion let's keep it simple considering Dr. Bach always intended flower essences to be for the layperson.

"No scientific explanation of how or why these remedies worked was offered by Dr. Bach. Indeed, he was wary of the "trends" that science is prone to, and encouraged others to keep his remedies "free from science, free from theories." If certain observable principles were operative in nature, there was no need to complicate the issue. Wild animals did not need an explanation of why certain plants helped them when they were ill." The Bach Flower Remedies, page X, first published in 1931 and in 1979 by Keats Publishing (New Canaan, CT).

Flower essence therapy began in 1930 with the British homeopathic physician, Dr. Edward Bach, noticing how he "felt" standing in front of a specific plant. For example, when standing in front of a mustard plant; he possibly felt depressed as this essence is used for depression. In front of gorse, he may have felt despondent as he said we should use this plant for hope. And so forth with his 38 remedies. Nowadays, I tell my students it is easier for our edification to first use a flower essence remedy and then discover how it makes us feel. Most of us are not as intuitive as was Dr. Bach.

St. John's Wort Personality

This yellow flowering plant I use for my flower essence is delicate and innocuous, not large in stature, less than 2 feet, but stands deliberate and erect. In full bloom, flowers and tendrils almost appear to twitch. I learned it is highly invasive and will "intelligently" travel underground deliberately emerging later at a great distance from its first planting.

The horse that may benefit from this plant is the one who may stand a bit taller in the head and shoulders, he may seem to do this deliberately and not be completely comfortable in this frame. Could be a bit on his toes. He may appear stoic, unengaged, following you with his eyes and not moving his body but, he knows exactly where you are and what your intentions are. If you move slowly around this horse; he will anticipate where you intend to touch and be more accepting in your approach.

Play with him. Hover your hand, barely cupped not flattened, a few inches above his fur and slowly, floating your hand over his body following a muscle contour or a line of some sorts. Spray your hands with essences, do the same thing, and see what changes in his bodily reaction. Are you invited in to be closer, work longer, make it a more enjoyable experience? That's the goal. Complements and other essences for this type are passion flower, lavender, and iris. Lavender essential oil is nice for this personality. Maybe invite them to lower their heads, softening the throat latch, relieving the neck and shoulders which relaxes the back and on through the topline until the entire body is comfortably affected.

Lobelia Personality.

Extreme cases can't bear to be touched. Tolerating the softest brushes and chamois but just does not enjoy being touched. Either they are literally thin-skinned or their hypersensitive nervous systems prevent them from enjoying human touch. Not to be confused with the avoidance behaviors of the abused horse or the one suffering actual physical pain. Respiration is superficial, never seeming to take in a big breath or fully exhale. They tend to lean forward slightly with an expectation to be hurt or made to feel uncomfortable. They may stop eating or drinking when you are around. They tend to have very expressive eyes often showing a worrisome confusion or concern, and may perspire on the face showing mental and emotional discomfort.

Historically, lobelia was used as a nerve tonic for humans and as a special ingredient in love potions. So, here I say, allow this personality to fall in love with you. Create a comfortable space of safety for them to enter when in your presence. If they tend to lean forward a few inches in a protective stance; you lean back. Take an actual step back, if you need, in order for them to want to approach you. Give this horse time, space and lobelia flower essence. Complements and further support are essences of rose and impatiens.

Sweet Pea Personality

Use sweet pea essence when you need "round-the-clock kindness." This personality wants to be kind and gentle but it takes great effort on their part. Touch with kindness, gentleness, but with determination.

Don't mislead or lie to this type. Once trusted; don't change the game plan. These horses tend to be flighty and nervous ready to evade or evacuate at a moment's notice. They are insecure and vulnerable but often behave contrary in order to protect themselves.

Nasty and unfriendly for no apparent reason, often nicknamed a witchy mare, even if it is a gelding. I had a mare like this; she would dictate my mood just by the way she was standing on any given morning. She seemed always ready for a fight or a flight to the extent that her feet more hovered over the ground than connected to it.

Riding The "Don't Touch Me" Horse

Sweet pea types can be a challenge to ride as we need to trust and relax enough to discover their rhythm, their stride. Try to make every effort to make them feel safe and secure. If necessary, ask a friend with a trustworthy mount to help as a companion rider, building self-reliance and self-esteem while making them feel they are part of the solution and not the problem. Complements for sweet pea horse and rider are apple, dandelion, and red clover essences.

St. John's Wort horses should be ridden quietly aware of every twitch and tingle. Can you feel him getting taller? Where does the sweat begin? Face, forehead, large muscle groups, the legs? Have you found their "sweet spot" while working with them on the ground? Withers, neck, shoulder? Using your creativity, discover how they will learn to trust, be more comfortable, and accept new challenges. Use your flower essences before, during, and after your time together until the need is no longer there.

Lobelia types are amazing to ride because they are so sensitive. Reins can simply be opened to create a place of safety for them to move into, arching into the openness and following with the nose—contrary to most riding styles. Opening your leg acts on them the same way, allowing them to close the gap intentionally. Pulling up your knee and hip just a few inches, gently moves your lower leg. This movement engages the entire midsection of the body with the resulting effort balanced and graceful. Same premise as a back without a perfect topline.

We don't add padding under the saddle to fill in the depressed areas; instead, we create space to encourage the topline to comfortably move up into.

Contrary to what I have possibly implied; these ultrasensitive animals are my favorites to work with and ride. They are honest and communicative, not misleading. Instructions and requests often have to be repeated and if not well received, don't push, give them a treat with their essences and put them up. Do some impatiens essence and start fresh at a later time.

Mist flower essences over the body and down the legs, and under the belly. Avoid eyes, genitalia, any open wounds, and bare skin. Spray your grooming equipment, use in bath water, drinking water, or food. Spray your hands for touch and massage. Also, think about spraying your hands before picking up your leadropes and leashes for time spent together.

Basic Training with Trust and Co-operation

Dr. Edward Bach, the 1930's British homeopathic physician and discoverer of Flower Essence remedies, wrote: "The action of these remedies is [...] to flood our natures with the particular virtue (def: good results) we need, and wash out from us the fault which is causing harm." To conquer a fault or a wrong requires steady development of the opposing virtue (good result), not suppression of the fault.

What Flower Essences Can Do

Flower essence remedies transform problematic behavior, attitudes, emotions, and patterns of learning, allowing anyone to excel to his or her fullest potential. They offer not just success on obvious behavioral or emotional situations but long-term, permanent solutions to even chronic problems.

There is no substitute for patience, training and understanding but sometimes we simply need to pull the lamp closer to get a better look—at ourselves as well. Flower essences illuminate, allowing us to see from a different angle, giving us an opportunity to reflect and make a long term change. Whether dealing with an excessive personality trait, an ingrained fear or a brand new experience, remedies can give us that moment of opportunity to make IT work—whatever our IT is at the time.

Flower Essences Help during Training

Years ago, I was hired to gentle 4 Thoroughbred colts who had never been handled because they were going to be race horses and the owners thought wild was the way to go. When I walked into the pasture, they rushed me, coming so fast and so close that I scrambled over the top of the fence to safety. I put 10 drops of Angels' Trumpet for trust, Cherry Plum for control, Impatiens for patience, Rock Rose for courage, and Star of Bethlehem for inner-peace into the 400-gallon water trough. When I returned the next day, same thing happened and they rushed toward me, but stopped in a cloud of dust 20 feet in front from me, lowered their heads, and slowly approached to within arms' length. One came closer and let me touch his nose. This colt had all 4 feet trimmed within 90 minutes of accepting his first halter. This proved a wonderful combination of essences, helping to establish trust for long-term relationships.

In training, some behaviors we request are complicated for the animal and require a series of adjustments to execute. Flower essences can help with these adjustments by encouraging a particular behavior or understanding from your animal. For example, Chestnut Bud and Clematis are integral to focus, learning, and acceptance of the procedures. Tiger Lily is for encouraging a team spirit in the horse and rider.

Training tips:

My opinion is that every time we handle a horse we are training. Every day, we have the chance to improve the horse-human relationship. How can we do this?

—One of the most important things we can do as a "trainer" is learn to apologize. I had ridden, taught and trained for 25 years before I realized how far down the road a simple apology would get me and my horses. Gentian is the essence I use for this since in homeopathics this is a wonderful remedy for "matters of the heart" and in essence form, I believe it helps courage and optimism replace doubt and pessimism. Also, Arnica essence is for cleansing hurtful memories, Gorse is for hope, and Mimulus is for known fears. Damaged and traumatized horses do well on this combination. This combination gives horses and humans a fresh start.

—In training procedures, we can create a positive atmosphere by vigilantly looking for the TRY. Most horse people are used to big deals, and unless there is drama, flair and a bit of the unnatural, some are not satisfied that ENOUGH has happened.

—We all benefit from having a basic plan, whether it is for the next 15 minutes or the next three weeks. And, just in case, I always have a "plan B".

—Avoid setbacks by giving essences in advance. For example, trailering presents its own set of problems, best avoided from the first time a horse is introduced to the trailer. To avoid negative reactions in the first place, use the remedies for trust and acceptance. Trailers to some horses are very scary, loud, dark and full of unnatural movement. Arnica essence is used here for security, Impatiens and Cherry Plum while taking a few extra minutes in the beginning to help adjust, and Clematis for focus and learning through experience.

Overcome Past Issues with Flower Essences

Horses are incredible one-time learners, not always for the best. One bad experience (like trailering) can prove difficult to overcome but it is possible to get a horse to overcome the fear or phobia. Use Mustard for anxiety caused by external circumstances, Mimulus for known fears, Star of Bethlehem for recovery from previous trauma or shock, and Star Tulip for grounding and creating a new experience.

During the process of change, a myriad of behaviors can surface. Be ready for this and address each one as it appears, and proceed. Rescued and re-habbed animals generally suffer through this because there is so much baggage to their lives. Typically, as they are made comfortable in their new surroundings and begin to relax and trust, their issues manifest and surface, and begin to create chaos in their new ordered world. Patience and understanding of their circumstances while using essences will get most animals right again.

Choosing and Evaluating Essences for Your Horse

Observation is the best judge when it comes to selecting which essences or blends to use, and when. If we observe the horse, noting his personality and its difficulties, we can see how he uses his brain, body and personality to (mis)behave, and we can choose suitable essences.

If progress is slow or personality flaws still exist, ask yourself: Was it the appropriate remedy in the right dosage and frequency? Is there a physical ailment or limitation that needs to be addressed by a health care professional? Are there any mental deficiencies that prevent the animal from working and thinking at his maximum? Has the best possible environment been provided? Was the desired result possible? With this animal? Within this environment? Most difficult to answer: was there change and you missed it or it was not the one you were looking for but the one that the animal needed? Do you need to modify your expectations? Do you need to see if you are part of the problem? These are tough questions, but don't be afraid to ask.

We and our animals can improve our relationships by overcoming the "faults that cause us harm". We can replace those faults by simply developing good results, naturally, with the help of flower essences.

Part Three—Making Sure You Are Not The Problem

Fix Yourself First

Owners Beware

Be aware of your power to influence your animals' behavior—for better or worse. I used to tell my students: Every time you handle your horse, you are training... where he stands when you open the gate, how he passes through the gate, grooming, tacking up, and riding. A related important suggestion is: If you are not feeling 100%, and not at your personal best, don't handle your horse. Why? They pick up on everything. Everything. Sure, *we* might feel better after being with them, but how are *they* at the end of our time together? Confused? Tired? Ready to be left alone for awhile?

If you are not at your best, then sit down and hang out. Figure out what your problem is and take care of it. Do your flower essences. Are you worried about bills? Mimulus is excellent for known fears. Are you fighting with your family? Figure out your part in it by taking some Clematis essence to expose your part in the misunderstanding. Don't daydream through a difficulty. Depression is rampant these days with all the bad news in the world. Mustard is for lingering depression that keeps coming back day after day. Dandelion is for depression that seems to have settled into your bones, exhausting you, depleting your innate courage. Aconite is an answer for sudden bad news.

What I am really saying here is don't worry about your animals until you fix yourself—before you inflict damage on them. If there is existing emotional or mental damage in the animal from previous experiences or events beyond our control, then use essences to address the damage. It does not matter how long ago the experience happened. One Australian Shepherd, Daisy, witnessed—from her apartment window—the Twin Towers coming down on 9-11 in New York City. She was alone. Her guardian had to walk home 2 miles amid debris and chaos arriving late in the afternoon to a traumatized dog. Ever since that day, Daisy reacted to loud noises, thunderstorms, and traffic by going to the window, staring outside and trembling. Her guardian gave her Sweetgrass essence for welcoming change, Gorse for re-newed hope, Yarrow for environment and homeopathic Aconitum 30x for shock. Daisy stopped her fear-based shaking, switched her focus to her guardian, and had no more trembling episodes.

Mirrors and Escalators

Did you ever notice that when you are having a bad day, so is your horse? It's not a coincidence. It is a mirror. They reflect our frustrations and impatience. A veteran horsewoman once advised: "If your horse is not understanding what you are asking of him, stop and put him up for the night." This went against everything I knew about "never give in or they will be spoiled". But she has been proven right dozens of times. I once was schooling a 3-year-old Paint mare who was not understanding my request for a side pass. I got off her, pushed her, got on, used heel, rein, and scratched her shoulder so she would move away from the pressure. NOTHING. Actually the harder I tried, the worse the whole thing became. I remembered what the older trainer told me and stopped. Reluctantly, I dismounted, gave the mare a reward and ended the lesson for the day. In that reward was Impatiens essence for patience, Mimulus if any fear arose during the session, and most important, Chestnut Bud.

Dr. Edward Bach wrote in *The Twelve Healers* about Chestnut Bud essence: "For those who do not take full advantage of observation and experience, and who take a longer time than others to learn the lessons of daily life." (*The Twelve Healers* published in 1931 by CW Daniels Co. Ltd., London. Re-printed in 1977 by Keats Pub., Inc New Canaan, CT under the name "The Bach Flower Remedies" quote from page 97.)

The next day, she was excited to work. I thought it was because I had quit the previous lesson early but after her warm-up, she took one awkward step without being asked, so I corrected her. But she did it again. Lo and behold, I gave her a loose rein and she started sidepassing. She stepped to the side with ease, grace and balance. I asked her to sidepass in the opposite direction and she performed with the same grace and balance, nothing I could have achieved in weeks of pushing myself on her. The day before, she was confused, which created frustration for us both, escalating negative emotions and behavior and thus heading us straight for anger. Chestnut Bud is my favorite for these situations.

Trade Up

I recently visited a place where I thought negative emotions would be running rampant, our local therapeutic riding center. I expected negativity because of the emotional burden and stress of families living with a disabled or challenged person. To my surprise, every single person, rider, sibling, caregiver, instructor, volunteer, and every horse appeared content and happy while caring for each other. Emotional transfer at its best.

In this day and age of bad news and focus on all things negative, the afternoon spent watching miracles rejuvenated my faith in mankind.

It was an incredible shout-out for the horses and the part they play in these children's therapy. In 90 minutes, I saw 2 young people who were never expected to walk, talk, or sit up. Both were not only able to talk, walk and sit up—they rode horses! How can hope have a limit? Positive emotions transferred from the horses and environment to the riders and their families = priceless.

Neutralize Emotional Disturbances in Companion Animals

Think about every horse you've had or who's had you. Your top two complaints probably boiled down to phrases like: I can't catch him. He is aloof. He doesn't hang out with me when he is at liberty. Or from the too-close side of life: He didn't mean to step on my foot. It was an accident. He head-rubs me because he likes me.

If you look closely at the behavior and its rewards for the equine, "too far" and "too close" appear to be opposite sides of the same coin. And for all intents and purposes, they are. But the same exact essences will help these seemingly different behaviors.

Too Far—*Aloof*
This is probably the most disturbing to me personally. I want to be friends with my horses, whether I am with them one hour a week or am living with them. Plus a herd animal, in its perfect condition, is not separate from the others. So I go poking around, trying to discover the reason for this odd behavior. I take inventory, asking questions and ruling out physical ailments and injuries. Are they depressed? Out of sorts? Got their feelings hurt? Did anything in the herd change recently? New additions? Did someone leave? Change of status in the herd?

Bonding with a human is not the most natural act for an equine even though we have been crawling on their backs for thousands of years. In my eyes, bonding is different from dependence (for food, water, shelter) and is different from human imprinting at birth. Historically, my experience has been that imprinted horses have little emotional interaction with no respect for others' space—human or equine. These horses tend to be pushy and/or leaners (lean on the hooftrimmer or lean on you). Is it that they don't know how to be friends? Lack socialization from mother and herd? Whatever the cause, flower essence therapy will establish balance in these personality extremes.

The bonding I am talking about is much more about trust— simple things like not stepping on my foot EVER, not knocking me down EVER, getting me home safely EVERY TIME. These simple requests have been hard won at times on difficult, aloof horses. Those personalities seem to not be in the "here and now" and, sorry to say, that does make them dangerous. They "wake up" and over-react.

Too Close—*Pushy*

Bossy, domineering, insecure, and afraid—equally distressing for the caregivers, riders, and handlers—are all on the other side of the coin. In the majority of my experience, aggression is fear-based. And fearful horses are dangerous in their attempts to flee or protect themselves, and may overreact to what they fear.

Change Can Happen

Bullies and victims actually benefit from the same flower essences, because the essences restore emotional balance. Somewhere in the middle of theses extremes is where a horse wants to be—a mentally, physically, and emotionally balanced member of the herd. Flower essences help him get there, and stay there. Even in the balanced horse, on any given day, change can happen, for better or for worse, in the blink of an eye. Maybe the wind blows the tarp off the hay, the farrier arrives in a bad mood, or there is an unavoidable change in the feeding schedule. Address such changes using the same essences used for chronic problems.

No Excuses

Stop giving excuses for potentially dangerous behaviors, and don't create such bad habits in the first place. Head rubbing, for example, I call hit-and-run. It is not a sign of friendship as most would have us believe. This is no way to communicate friendship.

Case in point: I had a client with a QH/TB named Max who would go out of his way to rub his head on his human, John, who was 6'3" and 240 pounds. Max would actually pick John up off the ground and move him around. The next day, little me showed up with 2 flakes of hay in my arms. I got tossed around with the force he'd used on John. Inappropriate; bad manners; reinforced negative behavior because John considered head rubbing 'bonding'. Truth of the matter is John was being pushed around by Max and Max treated all humans the same, until flower essence therapy showed Max that 'pushy' isn't necessary and John showed Max that 'pushy' is not desired. John got it too—in his water! We can use the same remedies for bullies and victims alike because flower essence therapy neutralizes emotional disturbances.

Remedies

Here are the solutions for getting and keeping horses focused in the "here and now" whether working at liberty, riding, trailering or standing calmly for a practitioner.

Pine flower essence helps in becoming aware of your surroundings in a grounded, calm, accepting manner, rooted" where you are—not in a stubborn, rigid way but more about growing strong where you are planted. Dried needles are actually best. I discovered this when the stickiness got in the way of creating an essence one afternoon. Also when making Pine essential oil, dried needles are used instead of fresh. How convenient for the planet! One more thing about using Pine flower essence—observe the conscious contact the animals have with the earth after you use this essence. The stance is different. The cadence is different. This is a fun essence to observe and watch in action as the animal connects intentionally with each hoof.

Clematis flower essence is for that drifty, far-away quality. Clematis is a beautiful wispy flower of soft colors. Clematis not only helps with focus but to also take an active role in one's life, not being a helpless bystander without capacity to make decisions. Clematis is for those in need of stimulation, enthusiasm, and purposeful living.

Cherry Plum flower essence is appropriate if they give no warning before ill behavior, act impulsively without thought of self-preservation, or do something other than fight, flight or freeze, or do all of the aforementioned all at the same time! Some do not posture, nor hesitate, nor set themselves in a stance to protect themselves in the next erratic behavior; they have no control over their behavior. Cherry plum is for composure. In *A Practical Guide to Vibrational Medicine* by Richard Gerber, MD, Gerber writes: "Also for those who take unnecessary risks or act rashly, without thought for possible harm they might bring to themselves."

So when is a behavior too much? When it exceeds acceptable interactive behavior or becomes a potential danger to others. 'Good manners at all times' is one acceptable guideline—no more pushing anyone around, no head rubbing because neither are acceptable. If they start with this behavior after getting their tack off, grab a cloth and clean their faces! Feel free to put a few drops of Pine, Clematis, or Cherry Plum essence on it. Being one step ahead will ensure you don't get stepped on!

Encouraging Partnership

Intelligent disobedience is a term trainers use when animals do not follow known commands in light of the fact that this command is not the right course of action in this situation. For example, the companion dog for a sight impaired person is asked to cross the street when there is a car ready to turn into their path. The person hears the chirp from the light signal that it is safe to walk but the dog knows better.

I have totally given my horse his head and "quit riding" on more than one occasion including once when up to my stirrups in quick mud in Arizona, trouble jumping over 5' fences in New York, on the same trail as a Mountain Lion in California, sliding down shale hillsides in Arizona, and countless times in-between where the horse found safety for both of us. When I say I quit riding that does not mean I dismounted but, that is sage advice in certain situations. What I mean is I quit interfering with the horse by relaxing my legs, hands, and voice, while relying on his balance, his decisions to get us to safety.

Here is a good place to remind ourselves why we use flower essences: to improve and prevent problematic behavior, attitudes, emotions, and patterns of learning **because they go to the root cause of mental and emotional problems, not suppressing or masking the problematic behaviors to resurface later, as in later on down the trail.**

Pop quiz:

What weighs 13,230 pounds, is 80,000 years old, and covers 107 acres?

Answer: One Aspen Tree in Utah.

This particular tree called "Pando" appears to be a grove of 40,000 individual Aspen trees. In reality, it is one tree as every single trunk shares the exact same DNA stemming from one root system; thus making it one living organism. Not sure this is relevant to this article, but wanted to share this amazing demonstration from a tree that claims to be the oldest and largest living organism on the planet and we can use any leaf from any Aspen as an essence! All beings owe their existence to trees since without their ability to eliminate carbon dioxide and release oxygen— none of us would exist. Tree essences are about encouraging teamwork and co-operation resulting in predictable behaviors between partners.

Aspen

Aspen tree leaves, when used as a flower essence, are wonderful for fears where there is actually a trembling or physical response—just like the trembling of the Aspen leaf. This can be subtle and undetectable while other times appearing to paralyze the horse. This is called the freeze response of fight, flight, or freeze. When this fear strikes it is a form of shock and most often, their behavior cannot be trusted when they emerge from this "unconscious" state.

Trembling Aspen leaves indicate change in weather and give advance warning of approaching winds stirring up in an area. Composure and gentle acceptance of change is one benefit of using Aspen essence. Head tossing, lip slapping, and tail twitching usually are indicators of worse behaviors to follow and can be remedied with Aspen as well by addressing the root cause of these "twitchy" behaviors. Use for fears and nervous behaviors even when you are not exactly sure what the triggers are that will set off quaking behavior. Does not have to be evident in actual trembling as horses will often internalize fears. This repression can lead to exhaustion as their energy is spent in covering up what is really troublesome.

Back at home, use Aspen for those in need of deep rest. A time off for the truly exhausted personality always on high alert. This is a remedy I like to give and then leave them alone for deep, safe rest and relaxation. Good for lay-ups who have hyper-vigilant personalities to calm at a deep inner-level and restore emotional balance.

Birch

What I like about Birch is that the trees are hardy, highly adaptable, and found in groups, often isolated and independent, not relying upon large numbers to survive. This is the essence I would choose for the horse that appears to be reactive in a crowd. Use Birch essence for the one who does not think independently or listen to you at crucial times but goes with the crowd on every decision. This is a dangerous horse as he has given up self-reliance, independent thinking, and concern for your welfare automatically defaulting to herd flight mentality. Use this essence when you need your horse to pay attention to you and your requests. Co-operative connection with your horse is attainable using Birch.

Oak

Oak essence is used by personalities who drive themselves to exhaustion and ill health by an exaggerated drive to work hard, to be the leader—no matter what the personal cost. Oak is for the strong personality that can be a little bossy or pushy in trying to get his own way. This is not all negative as Oak personalities are true leaders and often do know what is best in a given situation. But we need to be able to "rein them in" in case they do not have all the facts to make a sound decision. The goal of using flower essences is to prevent possible mis-behaviors and remedy existing bad habits. Resisting the impulse to mis-behave—in this case, to always take the lead—makes for a safe, predictable, consistent ride.

Apple

Apple essence is my clear choice for the horse that needs a fresh image. Overcoming past mistakes and starting anew. I recommend using Apple tree essence because it is more accessible and has a longer blooming period than Crab Apple. Also, in my experience, Apple has a broader application in helping different personalities overcome difficulties. Apple encourages a fresh self-image resulting in greater self-acceptance and self-confidence.

As an essence, apple offers great potential to mature and grow into best version of self. Developing through responsible actions and reactions befitting the demands of their situation. Trustworthy—nothing more important than when you are hours away from home and "stumble upon" a difficult situation.

Use for recovery from negative experiences to eliminate the mental fear of possibly repeating the experience in the future. In the way arnica flower essence clears mental memories of a negative experience; apple essence cleanses doubt and untrustworthy, negative memories from the core of the heart.

Precautions and Prevention

Best advice I can offer after 55 years of loving horses: Know your horse. Know his limits. When part of a group, know the other horses and riders and their limits—don't be part of someone else's training session without your permission as this can be potentially dangerous.

Make sure your horse is listening to you and behaving as a partner before you set off on your ride. Sometimes, you may want to turn them out to run, buck, and roll before you get in the saddle. Some prefer to longe or work at liberty using this time to establish a positive relationship. And after your ride, moving at liberty, rolling, massage, hydrotherapy and using flower essences are good tools to prevent soreness and help prevent uncomfortable physical residuals on the next ride. I believe that warming up is equally as important as the cool down period for all exercise.

Spoiled—No Way, You Say

Jealous or Zealous?

While doing research for a client, I discovered the word *jealous* comes from the Latin word for *zealous*. This new fact made me take a look at what I had always observed to be "jealous" behavior, defined as: resentfully envious. Are jealous animals simply zealous (filled with eagerness/interest)? Or are they insecure? Spoiled? Trying to teach us a lesson? Or just plain crazy? (I'm kidding.)

Animals With(out) Human Emotions

Animals arrive in our lives without a written history explaining possible quirks, phobias, and negative behaviors. With limited vocabulary to explain confusing or complicated behaviors, we offer excuses for their excessive personality traits. Diagnosing emotional problems in animals has its limitations since we are restricted to imposing our vocabulary on them. The fancy word for this is anthropomorphism, defined as: attributing of human characteristics to gods, objects, animals, etc. In this vein, we tend to assign our limitations to the animals, emotional limitations including jealousy, pettiness, anger, possessiveness, etc.

Bo, the young Quarter Horse, loved me. He would look forward to my visits and the routine. My friend had several horses and we always followed the same order as to when, how, and where we worked them.

Bo was always first out of his paddock because he was the youngest and had the least patience. Routinely, the first thing I would do after arriving is grab his halter and hang my shirt on its hook. One day, I arrived and their retired police horse needed attention first, which changed our and Bo's routine. Following my routine, I hung my shirt on top of his halter.

We got the old horse comfortable and returned to get Bo out of his stall. His halter was there but my shirt was missing. Bo was always "at the ready" by the gate but, now he was outside in the corner of his turn-out. I'm not sure what I noticed first: the odd look on his face, or my muddy shirt in three pieces at his feet. He had thrashed, ripped and stomped on my shirt. The look on his face was half remorse and half triumph, as he knew he got his point across to us—Don't change the ordered routine, because it changes status.

Flower Essences to the Rescue

Star of Bethlehem flower essence is the absolute best for us and our animals since this essence is intended for shock, hurt feelings, confusion, and emotional experiences like getting bit, stepped on, or clawed—depending on your animal of choice. As I have previously written, it was the only single remedy that I took to the aftermath of Hurricane Katrina. One bottle went with a fellow volunteer to the hospital with a life-threatening spider bite returning for his second surgery. He asked me for it because he had witnessed the help it gave to hundreds of cats and dogs arriving daily from the floodwaters of New Orleans.

Star of Bethlehem is excellent for do-overs. The best example is when you need to apologize or back up the clock and re-address an incident. It's incredibly helpful for times when you do not know what happened but the animal is "off", a technical term for "don't have a clue as to what is wrong." It does not matter how long ago the incident happened; essences will help. If the transgression is recent, use essences more often, beginning with possibly every 10-15 minutes for the first hour and hourly for the next few hours until you see calm return to the animal. For chronic behavior or older incidents, use four times daily for a longer period of time, maybe a few weeks.

Blending Star of Bethlehem with Angel's Trumpet (used for self-empowerment) allows the animal the capacity to use discernment, judge a situation, and react appropriately. One owner said: "It gave him a pause button."

Tiger Lily essence can be used in cases where there is loss of status, insecurity, or difficulty believing in oneself. This essence provides a sophisticated focus encouraging learning and understanding while giving the animal a moment to change confusion, fear, or worry into mental and emotional confidence.

Indulged or Spoiled?

Whom should we pay attention to first? Whom should we feed first? The fastest and strongest, is my (safest) answer. Some believe the only answer is to give in to the negative behavior and its consequences, like smoothing riffs in the barnyard, calming nerves at feeding time, granting leniency, and giving excuses for crazy behavior when company arrives. I know people who rearrange furniture, schedules, and even vacation plans to suit their animals' idiosyncrasies and eccentricities.

I know there are fancier words than "pushy pigs" for dominant behavior but everyone can relate to the one cat that fights, growls and hogs the food. Or the horse pushing a shoulder into you or butting you with his head. And the dog who loves to play but always wants to be over the top of the other dog or stealing toys, and if reprimanded, usually wanders away with disinterest.

Normally, essences encourage better behavior within minutes or at most, after a few days of use. Severely damaged animals or chronic issues require more time but my experience is that permanent behavior improvement can be attained within one month. Blending essences of Red Clover to gently restore emotional balance, Gorse for hope, Sweet Pea for delicacy, patience, and kindness, and Mustard for lingering depression, in this case due to loss of family security, works wonders.

Plain Crazy? Maybe Not

Cats not letting someone into the inner-circle looks petty and cruel to us but it can also be that the new animal is sick, possibly with a transmissible disease threatening the entire "family" and the meanies are, in reality, protecting everyone by shunning this cat. Maybe we will never know the cause for the aggressive, negative behaviors but that does not mean we can't help them overcome their troubles and become contented, emotionally balanced individuals. If after giving flower essences a thorough try the animals still do not 'accept and get along', don't push it—just accept this and remember that these animals' innate intelligence has allowed them to survive upwards of 50 million years. If there is a reason or need for these behaviors in such circumstances, the essences won't override them (you can't fool Mother Nature).

Blending essences of Sweet Pea for kindness, Gorse for hope, and Mustard for lingering depression has worked wonders on many animals suffering from insecure dominance. Perseverance is necessary since we are changing an ingrained mental pattern not merely a bad habit. My experience is that flower essences will permanently improve behavior within one week of using a remedy. Then use if issues arise or you want to further improve behavior or advance training. In cases of mental damage from poor breeding practices and lack of proper socialization as youngsters resulting in negative behavior, it could take longer to temper the personality.

Even though I have been blending essences for 35 years, I still marvel at the powerful effectiveness and simplicity of it all. Here we are using plants in a form that is no fancier than a cup of tea but able to drastically improve lives. This time of year we can indulge our passion for flowers and create our own essences. Find your favorite (non-poisonous) flower, or weed in the case of Red Clover and Dandelion, place a few flower tops in a glass of water, set it in the sun for 20 minutes, and sip throughout the day. Not fancy. Simply powerful.

Another True Story about Bo's Love

A few weeks after Bo destroyed my shirt and taught me to stick with our routine; he again proved his love of his owner, "J". I was riding the old horse and "J" was riding Bo. This was a thrill for all because Bo was still so green and no one was sure his brakes would work in an emergency. We were in an open field and the wind started to pick up. And so did Bo's spirits. I asked "J" to switch horses with me. She hesitated. My concern about Bo's agitation grew to anger.

I said: "Give me the reins, now."

Standing there facing his shoulder with one leg bent at the knee angled out at 90 degrees, she said: "Mumble, mumble, please."

I said: "Now."

Waving her one foot behind her in the air, she said: "Leg up, please."

I said: "I want you to get away from Bo."

Again: "Leg up, please."

I certainly did not want her to get back on him. I wanted her to get away from this youngster before his behavior became reactive to my approaching horse, changing weather, and this greenhorn rider sucked up to his side. Then she slightly turned her head in my direction and said:

"I need a leg up. My bra is caught on the saddle."

Then I saw her boots were dangling in the air, inches from the ground. Her bra was wrapped tight around the saddle horn holding her up in mid-air. Bo stood while my horse and I approached and I lifted her bent knee up just enough to free herself and slide to the ground.

Bo was a perfect gentleman the entire time. He truly loved her. Imagine if it would have been me hung up like that? I could have ended up like my shirt ... with a matching bra.

Part Four—Best Friends from Beginning to End

A Soft Voice and a Light Touch
This advice is excellent for all introductions—not just birthing.

Our veterinarian arrived within 20 minutes and as we opened the ranch gates for him, he said, "Did I miss it? Sure hope not!" He was so enthusiastic at 2:00 in the morning that I had to ask how many foalings had he attended. His answer: "Somewhere around 6,000."

He first asked the mare's permission before entering her enclosure. He checked her and then quietly checked on the baby. He made sure the foal latched on to nurse, checked the placenta, and then leaned over the fence with the rest of us and just watched.

Richard Tramp, DVM and equine reproductive specialist in Valley Center, California gave us this advice when asked about further handling of this foal. "A light touch and soft voice is all she needs. Do that several times a day—start with Mama and ask permission to touch the foal."

Foalhood Flower Essences for All
We often presume that newborn foals have no issues, damage, or abuse. That may (or may not) be so, but upon birth, life on Earth—with all its challenges—begins. Fortunately there are some wonderful flower essences that welcome these beings into the world and help them cope with it. All these essences I will mention are as much or more for the humans as the foals. Make sure everything you use is diluted and in a soft misting spray bottle.

Impatiens essence, especially good for the humans, will give them patience to follow the timing of Mother Nature and not the clock. Sit back and enjoy the event!

Rose and Calla Lily are two essences that are very appropriate for birthings. Rose is the most incredible essence for being in the exact moment with trust, openness, and acceptance. Calla Lily, with its spiral flower, reflects hope and optimism. Sweetgrass is for welcoming change, appropriate for birthing. Yarrow is for environment, and if the foal (or anyone) appears stressed, sprinkle or mist some onto the ground.

Witchy Mares

A nasty, non-interactive mare can pass these traits down to the foal, so it is best if you can work with her in advance. Some sweet dispositioned mares become irritable, overly protective, and aggressive. Impatience, Red Clover, Sweet Pea, and Crab Apple are all wonderful for a stressful situation or dealing with a difficult person or animal.

Lavender essential oil (therapeutic grade) can be added to the essences mentioned above or dripped/ spritzed onto the stall door or near where visitors are going to be observing the birth and new foal. If the mare is extremely stressed, put a few drops on the wall near her feed or on the fencing where she stands, eats or drinks. Don't impose anything on her; let her decide. Even better is to spray yourself lightly and approach the mare. Be careful—hormonal changes can make her unpredictable.

Mistakes and Accidents

No matter how prepared we think we are, stuff happens. I know one foal who turned up at a neighbor's house… she had been born at night and rolled underneath the pipe corral, and once she stood up, she could not get back in to be with her mother. Also things such as doors slamming, tarps flapping, and dogs lurking around can all have devastating and lasting effects on babies.

Star of Bethlehem is the best remedy to help the foal "re-enter" the world from shock. If your foal has encountered any shocks like trailering, injury, or even being orphaned, Yarrow, Rock Rose, and Star of Bethlehem are perfect as singles or a blend. Remember, use them very diluted and gently misted in the air, or put some on your hands and gently massage in. Tips of the ears is a wonderful area to gently massage if they can handle that without adding to the stress.

Comfortable Correction

Passion Flower is a wonderful remedy if mistakes in handling have occurred and the foal's behavior has become unnatural or undesirable. This will gently guide the foal back to a more acceptable way of behaving. Gentian is for matters of the heart, so if you find that the youngster is owed an apology, use Gentian essence, for yourself as well.

Parting Can Be Sweet

Weaning methods are as controversial as any other subject with horse people. My observations are that to make a smooth, non-stressful transition it is best to wait for all the signs from the mother that she is ready to wean. Why rush it? Slow transition is safest. Move the mare but keep her close so that they can still see each other and hear each other, but not touch, for at least 3-5 days. Foals will try to crawl, jump or push their way back to the mother's side, so good safe fencing is immensely important for this separation. Then move her a bit further away when you see that the stress is not too great. This will prevent anger, fear, and trauma. Any of the above mentioned essences will be good to add to the water and feed upon weaning, depending on the baby's behavior.

It is essential that foals feel comfortable and secure in this world with humans and horses alike, so they can naturally adapt to life. They need to remain healthy and cooperative in the face of all challenges, relying on their natural instincts with the trust and respect they have for people and for their own kind. Flower essences work 100% of the time and they will help in any situation from birth, through training, and on to the "finished horse".

Aging With Comfort

Animals with us today, if given proper care, are living way into their golden years. But living to a ripe old age brings some special challenges.

From Edward Bach, M.D. and F. J. Wheeler, M.D. *The Bach Flower Remedies.* New Canaan, CT: Keats Publishing Inc., 1979:

> "... the new combination of elements that we use together are: 1) a physical diagnosis of a mental problem, 2) transmutation of feelings, 3) cementing with flower remedies, 4) and all the other available therapies such as homeopathic medicine, diet and nutrition, helping postural problems, fasting, and so on."

This solid plan of action is excellent if the behavioral problems are not exclusively mental, emotional, or personality difficulties. I would boldly say the elderly equine is in this category. So, use all information and resources available to provide the best life prognosis. Since flower essences do have a positive effect 100% of the time (when properly prepared and properly administered) and do complement every modality, use them with confidence while amending the difficulties troubling your horse.

1) A Physical Diagnosis of a Mental Problem

Helping the aging horse mentally and emotionally is only possible after ruling out possible physical causes that create the same troublesome behaviors. Cognitive Dysfunction Syndrome and equine dementia are two problems that need to be diagnosed with the help of a holistic veterinarian since the symptoms are virtually identical to the natural aging process.

Symptoms including aimless wandering, staring, head shaking, aggression, distractibility, and seizures (from simple eye flutters to fainting) could have physical origins since a number of diseases and disorders mimic symptoms of equine dementia. Common causes of these exact same symptoms and behaviors include parasites, worms, mites, fever, hormone imbalance, vitamin or mineral deficiency, exposure to mold, colic, heavy metal toxicity, and bug bites. Therefore, it is imperative to get a physical check up first before you assume the problem is solely due to aging.

Noting specific details of behaviors in an aging horse is important in order to provide the best care and not miss physical problems if they do arise later. Know your horse's daily and nightly habits, average temperature, heart rate, stomach sounds, drinking habits, and feeding schedule including how long it takes to finish a meal. Check on them during the day and late at night to notice any irregularities including sleeping patterns and/or difficulty in getting up. Do they stand there not moving for a while? Or do they move off immediately? This information will be your benchmark if habits and behaviors do change.

2) Transmutation of Feelings

Ruling out physical problems, we are free to take care of any negative behaviors ensuring best quality of mental health in the aging equine. Symptoms of depression tend to be first to manifest. Use single flower essence remedies or blends until you are able to give relief to the horse, his companions, and yourself. Aging is a (often rapid) progression and unfolds itself daily. Continually be alert for changes and re-address your selections accordingly.

Mild depression may be expressed as any of the following: less enthusiasm for favorite things (food, toys, companions), difficulty adjusting to new physical limitations, less focus, less patience, change in sleeping or napping habits, nervous agitation, and newly developed vices. Take care of the retiree who stands daily, staring as if waiting to be saddled and go for a ride, with Honeysuckle. Also, for this demonstration of unwavering devotion, use Rosemary essence. Sweetgrass essence is for accepting change, and Impatiens is used for increased tolerance and approval of the new situation.

Aggression associated with more severe depression is remedied with Rose flower essence. Equally effective is Passion Flower, a multi-faceted flower with soft tendrils, a will to flourish, and blooming for its own sake usually in adverse conditions. This flower will comfortably correct negative tendencies to act out, allowing the horse to calmly think of a more appropriate, positive response. Nasturtium is another flower that is excellent for restoring loss of dignity, eliminating confusion, and expressing the "normal" personality. "Normal" needs to be redefined in the older horse. What was once unacceptable behavior may be allowed, especially if that's all you get. Playing may take on a new dimension.

Unresolved grief is another possibility for negative behavior in the aging horse. Sudden changes, including retirement, can be traumatic as they represent a big change and may mean loss of identity as well as loss of status. Plus loss of time spent with you and that can easily lead to sadness. Maybe give them a new job or some way to engage their minds. Spray flower essences on safe toys, placed on the ground or hanging in the air, keeping their brains active and their bodies moving. Do something a little different to engage them positively. If their eyesight is compromised; bells and wind chimes can be used for directing to and distinguishing between water, food, and shelter. Companion animals can wear a bell to guide the sight-impaired animal.

3) Cementing with Flower Essences

Roses—for everyone. Rose flower essence is my #1 for aging animals and all of their friends. Make your own essence as follows: cut fresh, organically grown roses and float the flowers (whole or petals) covered with pure water in a glass bowl set in the sun for ½ to 1 hour. Strain and add the "solar-infused flower water" to drinking water, food, or bath water. Use while you massage and on grooming equipment. Make fresh every day.

Companions often feel the sadness and confusion of their aging friends. Treat these accordingly. However, some behaviors of the companion animals may appear uncharacteristic. For example, Chief, a 32-year-old Paint gelding lived for years in a pasture with several other geldings. They all got along and followed the hierarchy faithfully with Chief being respected as Alpha. One day, while Chief was trying to nap, 2 of the youngsters started picking on him. The young ones would not allow the old man to rest in peace. They circled Chief and appeared to bite his flanks. They got on opposite sides until Chief lifted his head.

They did not leave him alone until he was standing. Other times, they would chase him. At 32 years old, he was loaded with arthritic joints and a swayback, so that herd behavior appeared cruel until the vet informed me the youngsters were possibly trying to keep him alive by keeping him active. Later observations confirmed these actions were definitely acts of compassion for the old-timer.

Star of Bethlehem essence was given to Chief for restoring dignity. Rosemary essence is used to ease the effects of slower circulation including slower mental function. Use singly or combine with flower essences of Impatiens and Rose.

An aging horse often does better with a companion than living alone. Care needs to be taken that the new companion does not succumb to the same levels of inactivity and/or possible depression. Burn-out is possible if the aged horses take their caregiving position seriously. To prevent this, give them the same remedies plus give them regular time off from their caregiver's position before they get depressed or cranky. Vervain has been proven the perfect flower essence for those who are stoic, strong-willed, and overly self-confident. This type of Vervain personality, according to Dr. Bach in the aforementioned book: "In illness they struggle on long after many would have given up their duties."

Human counterparts suffering in heart-gripping sorrow are in need of Bleeding Heart essence. Our distress for the situation will have a direct effect on the comfort levels of our charges. To snap out of a negative state of mind, use Star of Bethlehem. Honeysuckle is perfect for disappointment. And, of course, help yourself to essences of Rose and Impatiens.

4) And All Other Available Therapies

Essential oils of Lavender, Rose, Rosemary, and Rose Geranium are excellent for geriatrics as they address anxiety, worry, and depression, and are best used separately. Allow the horse to choose what he wants. Put a few drops near feeding areas or water buckets. Be careful because oils will attract insects, including bees.

When Chief reached 34 years old, tests revealed he had only 5% kidney function. Euthanasia was suggested but I asked for 3 weeks. The vet started him on a round of antibiotics and I started him on flower essences and vegetable soup. Parsley, alfalfa, red clover, carrots with tops, dandelions, and other goodies simmered for an hour every day. We soaked his hay in this soup and fed it to him along with the mushy vegetables and flower essences. He loved it.

Moreover, he was given soothing sprays of flower essences all over his body. Twice a day, we put 10-20 drops of essences in 1 ounce of water (any of the ones mentioned in this article would be excellent choices) and generously sprayed him, paying special attention to the spine, base and tips of the ears, and massaging the gums liberally. If your horse really does not like a spray, apply with a sponge, dandy brush, or piece of cloth. 3 weeks later, Chief's blood work showed normal kidney function. The vet gave credit to the antibiotics while I gave credit to the herbs and essences. He died a year later due to heart failure in his pasture full of friends.

As you age with your horse, keep in mind, and foremost in your heart, that you are the one who best knows your best friend. Learn your choices. Find advisors you trust. Work within your budget. Address every day as unique and adjust to changes accordingly.

Living Beyond Grief

"Grief is any distressing emotion or behavior that arises out of a change," according to Sandy Heath, certified grief recovery counselor in San Diego, California.

Horses love consistency and routine and may react strongly when that is upset for any reason. Separation from a loved one or a lifestyle change can create irreconcilable feelings of insecurity and unfamiliarity.

Grief in horses can appear as depression, anger, anxiety, impatience, or any multitude of behaviors. Of course, this is normal for any loss or change but if the horse has not gotten better within a given period of time, then attitude and behavior can be affected with long-term negative consequences.

Essences for Grief

Flower Essences are extremely helpful in times of grief. They do not take away from the experience but enhance recovery. Depression and despondency with failure to thrive can be observed through loss of appetite, drinking less, gloom in all undertakings, and most often the eyes change, no longer reflecting a world that is hospitable. Change has overwhelmed them.

Star of Bethlehem is my single most important remedy, and I am seldom without it—I carried several bottles to the Gulf Region post-Katrina. I use this essence for shock and trauma, no matter how long ago the experience. This is the remedy that gets immediate results for me when the horse just cannot cope and is acting poorly.

Oak and Mustard essences are wonderful for overturning depression and despair. Oak is for exhaustion from trying to be strong. Mustard is used when horses appear to be giving up and not participating with their former enthusiasm. Mustard is good for those who feel resigned to the fact they have no control over their lives.

Saying Good-Bye

A wonderful Quarter Horse mare came to us as a rescue. We got her sound and loved her dearly for many years. She babysat my six-year-old son and was smooth as silk with him in the corral or on the trail.

While playing in the pasture, she tore all the ligaments and tendons away from her knee tripping in a gopher hole. The vet said she had a 50/50 chance. We did everything we could for her for the next 18 months. I had made a promise that I was never going to give up on her, until I saw what would change my mind. She was playing in the pasture with our other horses when she pulled herself out of the game, went behind a tree and hung her head in pain. I knew then that her quality of life would force the worse decision any horse owner will ever have to make.

Euthanasia in Greek means "good death" and I have come to believe it is an inherent responsibility that follows domestication. I have learned that it is never the perfect answer, that there is never a good time, and that I've never been 100% certain in any of the 11 times that I have had to make the decision. I have rescued so many horses in my lifetime and been incredibly successful re-habilitating them and placing them in good homes, but the reality is that not all are going to make it.

I did not let Pony and our Clydesdale-Thoroughbred, Bubba, say "good-bye" to their stable mate when she left. I thought I was doing the right thing but Bubba told me different—he was immediately angry and agitated, and he bucked me off every time I rode him for the next three weeks. I wanted him to go through the grieving process in his own time, but he was stuck—and I was on the ground way too much—so I intervened.

I gave him Gentian flower essence, which is for matters of the heart. He also received Gorse for hope and his loss of trust. The world had changed and was no longer in its proper order. Rock Rose is a good essence for this behavior, addressing panic and uncertainty, giving the horse a chance to quiet down and accept the new situation.

Other Grief Instances that Benefit from Essences

Destructive behaviors are sometimes easier to treat because you can address the behaviors, but if the animal has shut down, then the task is more difficult. Some live with a kind of quiet desperation and the blend of essences to turn that around is Mimulus for known fears, Star Tulip for grounding, Rock Rose for suppressed panic, and Angel's Trumpet for incorporating the new awareness and change. Also, Forget-Me-Not is wonderful and gentle for these types of behaviors.

My son worked as a vet tech in an equine hospital and has told me the majority of colic cases are because the horse experienced a sudden change in feed, water source, environment, or exercise routine. Helpful essences are Yarrow for environment, Star of Bethlehem for shock, Star Tulip for grounding, and Sweetgrass for accepting change.

Starr was a horse I wrote about previously who was traumatized by abuse and neglect and became extremely dangerous. What I did not write in that article is that she had seriously injured two people before she came to stay with me. The owner told me that the mare attacked his wife sending her to the hospital with a broken foot because she "… watered the mare at the wrong time." This may sound like an extreme example but horses that are confused, hurt, or insecure are unpredictable and therefore can be dangerous.

Moving can be stressful.

I used to take it personally if horses did not settle in at my farm but then I came to realize maybe they missed their herd or that they were confused and concerned about their place in the new herd. For these feelings of settling into a new environment, I use Dandelion for courage, Yarrow for environment, and Arnica for acceptance.

According to the grief recovery counselor: "We never intentionally inflict our negative emotions on our animals but sometimes they pick up on them and "absorb" our depression and grief." If that has happened, use any of the previously suggested essences—especially Gentian, which is great for apologizing.

Some losses seem impossible to accept with the feeling we will never get beyond the difficult emotions and the weight of our grief. If that is the case, Bleeding Heart is incredible for healing the broken heart. Again, with essences, time does not matter. Use Bleeding Heart or the others mentioned here to recover from losses inflicted decades earlier. It will work for you and those you are trying to help.

Making Sure You Have the Right Answers is as Easy as 1, 2, 3

#1 is the opportunity of listening to others for advice.
#2 is information about the "science of applied kinesiology" and how it applies to you.
#3 is some good books.

I have been interested/obsessed with traditional care for 40 years. In the early 1970's, I asked a book store employee where I might find books on 'healing with herbs' and she told me to check in the "occult" section. (An herb is defined as any plant ever used for its medicinal, savory, or aromatic qualities—that's all.) What I hope for from this book is to bridge a bit of the gap that still exists from getting the plants to animals.

We, and I am included in this population, continue to have nagging doubts and worry that these alternatives really do not work and there is delusion in the air. Then, I have one more "aha" moment with one more "aha" animal as it reveals its true personality and innate lovingness to me when those films of negative memories and experiences are "melted like snow in the sunshine," as Dr. Bach once wrote.

#1. Listening to learn. Learning to listen.

Neither one comes easily to me. We have a generation or 2 coming up that are easier to listen to concerning their innate knowledge of plants and animals. These youngsters don't need to go through years of doubt and validation and more doubt. These "kids" have a comfortable acceptance that we are closely related with the world and there is a need to foster that relationship. There are many making wise personal choices and studying natural remedies in school including ethnobotany—the study of plants helping man. Remember Imo the young Monkey was first to wash her sweet potato and then taught her Mother. Listen to the young ones.

SIERRA AND THE DIXIE CUPS is not a band but one young woman with a mission. Sierra was 9 years old when I went to her house one day and saw Dixie cups all over the yard and up the porch steps. When I looked into the paper cups, I saw flowers in water. Each cup had a different flower. Sierra was making her own Essences. She made her choices based on her intuition and her feelings about the flowers. She made wonderful Essences. Very powerful. Some older people are now coming aboard the band wagon and soaking up this knowledge and experimenting. If there is one message—it is to not take any of this too seriously and just PLAY.

#2. Testing for All.

Muscle Testing: A DIAGNOSTIC TOOL for all ages.

Muscle testing, the science known as Applied Kinesiology, is a simple process whereby the body actually gives answers, physical signs of what is "good" for it at any particular time. For our purposes, we want to obtain answers concerning the needs and overall well-being of any person or animal, getting a "yes" or a "no" response as to whether "***something***" is #1 beneficial for "***someone***," #2 in what quantities, and #3 for what duration.

My first instruction in kinesiology was in Chicago in 1970. The book was mimeograph papers—remember how good that ink smelled?—bound by plastic. The pictures were amateurish and the type too big. But it was the new science and I wanted to learn it. Class was held on a Saturday at a medical office on prestigious Michigan Avenue. I asked about classes available during the week and got a shocked NO from the doctor explaining he did not want his colleagues seeing him instruct such an un-scientific science.

After 40 years, I am extremely comfortable with muscle testing and the answers afforded me. And grateful for the answers denied me. This is not a divination game. You will not get lotto numbers or the amount of next month's bank statement. How do I know? Never mind.

Certain doctors and practitioners, meticulously trained in this applied science, excel at diagnosing and prescribing for individuals from the body's own indisputable responses. What I am about to explain is for the everyday person from a layperson with 40 years practicing different methods specializing in animals.

FOR BEST RESULTS: No cell phones, etc. & no cigarettes & no wallets on either person, as any of these can skew results. No crossed legs, arms or fingers. Simple.

THE PARTNER METHOD

1. Get a partner.

Ask if there are any physical limitations. Old injuries? Arthritis? Soreness anywhere? If yes: try one of the other methods listed below. If all clear; proceed.

PERSON #1 With feet flat on the ground and one arm hanging at your side, raise the other arm straight in front of your body with hand (palm down open flat) shoulder height.

PERSON #2 Put two fingers on the top of your partner's raised wrist while keeping your elbow straight while gently (3-5 pounds pressure—no more) pushing that arm down toward the floor while asking questions. Try not to stand directly in front of each other while testing.

Begin asking questions requiring YES or NO responses:
What is _____'s (name of person) YES today?
What is _____'s NO today.

➢ Don't fluctuate pressure. Don't fluctuate resistance.

➢ Holding strong is a YES response. Re-test to be sure.

➢ Unable to hold arm straight in front of the body is a NO.

➢ NO is demonstrated as a few stubborn inches or total weakness in the arm.

➢ Change arms when one becomes tired and avoid over-testing in one session.

Before going further—make sure you are able to get clear, definitive answers—as this is important to every question you ask. Here's an exercise:

Ask for an obvious YES such as the person's name. Or ask for a NO. Make up a name and ask: "Is your name Puddin' Tane?" Don't dwell on the negative but asking for a drastic NO will generate discernible answers obvious to both partners.

Ask: "Is this product (cigarettes, soda, candy) good for _____so-and-so_____?" Even better, see if there is a cigarette, soda or candy bar and have the person hold it close. Results are obvious.

This works on skeptics (including teenagers and spouses) every time—guaranteed. Never want to go too negative but sometimes it is necessary when the personality in front of you is being particularly obstinate or stubborn.

2. **Testing a Product.**

Following above instructions and now Person #1 holds any product with "free" hand close to their chest. Either person can ask the questions while GENTLY applying the <u>same, consistent amount of pressure</u> in a downward motion to the top of Person #1's wrist.

If the product is NOT beneficial to the individual at this time: the arm will lower. Don't fight or try to overpower each other. This is a gentle yet firm test and the results are unmistakable. Some only bend a few inches while others crash the arm to their side. Most are somewhere in-between these extremes. But NO is NO.

3. Questions to Ask

If you are getting a YES response for a certain product; now ask:

A. <u>How many drops or sprays?</u> Count one, two, three, four, five… Whenever you weaken—that is too much. So if at four you are strong and you weaken at five; then the dose is four drops.

B. <u>How often?</u> Once a day, twice a day, three times a day… If you weaken at five; then four times a day is the frequency.

C. <u>How?</u> Ask and wait for individual response. In water? Food? On the body?

How many days? or How many weeks? One, two, three… Re-test every day—just to be on the safe side.

WOO-WOO TRAIN… Next stop… Animal Testing… All Aboard…

4. You can get answers for any animal.

First, get a YES and NO answer from your partner. Initially say: Testing for _____ (name of the person holding their arm out).
What is _____ YES today?
What is _____ NO today? Get a definitive response for both positive YES and negative NO.

Second, say: Testing for _____ (use real name of the animal.)
What is _____ YES today?

What is _____ NO today? Get a definitive response for both positive YES and negative NO.

Third, when this response is obvious for a YES and a NO; have your partner hold the product on or close to the animal, and proceed with questions C. 1-4 as above.

5. What if the animal is not accessible? Too aggressive to approach, too far away, or an emergency situation exists. Simply, hold the product yourself and follow above explanation in step 4, establishing definitive responses for the animal you want to test. Then ask same questions: #3. A-C. You will see definitive answers.

As you get comfortable with muscle testing, you can also ask questions about food, water source, care, equipment, supplements, quantities, etc. Remember: Make certain questions asked have simple YES and NO answers. Re-test often.

GOING-IT-ALONE METHODS

In the real world, we don't always have the luxury of having a partner present. Here are several methods for those times. Before testing, ask: What is my YES today? What is my NO today? They will often vary day to day, depending on the time of day, where you are standing, and the direction you are facing. Trust me (and trust my mistakes and misunderstandings) that responses do vary and this is an important step for accurate information.

When you have established your YES and NO responses for yourself and your animals; then choose from any of the following methods; hold the product, and ask questions listed above as: #3. A, B, C.

The Sway Method

Stand comfortably with feet a touch apart. Eyes open or closed. Arms loosely at you sides.

Ask: What is my YES today? Wait. Wait. Wait. Wait until your body slightly leans in one direction. Forward. Backward. One side. Or the other. Few people actually feel themselves swirling in a small circle. Clockwise. Counter-clockwise. Some drastically move in one direction or another and have to put out a foot to steady themselves. Some do not move at all.

Ask: What is my NO today? Wait. Wait. Wait. Moving? Nothing? Some individuals move ever so slightly in one direction or another and that is their answer, their NO. Try with eyes closed and ask again. If you get a movement in your YES and nothing for your NO—that could be the demonstration of your NO = NO movement.

For demonstrable effects: ask if this is Wednesday or Saturday. Or ask: Is my name Fluffy? Play with this method. Stand facing different directions and see if there is any variation. Movements are often quite dramatic. While others do not respond at all, if so; try another method.

The Head Nod

Exact same as above but just move your head. You can be seated—in a crowded room—at Dog Park—even in the saddle—and no one will have any idea what you are up to unless you are the "whiplash type." Personally, I am a head snapper. I look like I'm doing the Funky Chicken dance from 1964. But it's effective.

Circles of Fingers

This one is difficult for me as I feel the response is not definitive enough and I get tired snapping my hands apart several times. But that's just me and actually this method is very popular.

Bring together thumb and index finger in a perfect circle—nails touching if necessary. Same with the other hand but close the circle inside the other fingers' circle. Like a link. Or a figure 8 intertwined.

YES is when you pull apart while asking a question and the circles remain strong—fingers do not separate.

NO is when the chain breaks apart—fingers break open. Unless you can THINK about the product and get accurate results; this method forces you to put the product under your arm or in your pocket to test—I find it awkward.

One-Handed

This is the one I use a lot. Place middle finger on top of index finger. End of middle finger is on top of nail on index finger. That is where and how you apply pressure to receive your answers—by pushing slightly "down" on top of index finger trying to make it bend.

YES is when you ask a question and your index finger remains strong.

NO is when you can push you index finger "down" slightly bending it at middle knuckle.

The Rub

My wonderful Girlfriend showed me this just last year and it's great. The gist of it is simply rub your index finger and thumb together. Like you had Elmer's glue or rubber cement and it was fun to gently roll it in a ball between your fingers.

YES is all circuits go and you can rub the tops of these 2 fingers either in a circular or back-and-forth motion all day long.

NO is when movement stops, similar to a sticky feeling. My fingers actually slide off from each other and stop. Alisa's actually get sticky. She says it feels like her fingerprints rise. One person said his "fingertips sweat." LOTS OF FUN TO TRY. Has turned out to be my newest favorite method especially for students just beginning.

With these practices, anyone, anywhere, can work on horses, dogs, cats while others have no idea what you are up to. While talking to someone, put your hand behind your back or just dropped to your side, and then "check on" or "ask" about animal's food, absorption, water source and consumption or problems they may be encountering. Ask: Is this animal properly hydrated? Is his food nutritious? Need something else in his diet? Any etcetera for any animal you think will help the quality of their lives.

Pendulums users are comfortable with the answers they receive. My ONLY problem is what if you need it and realize you left your object in your other coat pocket. Then what? Pendulum users: try one of these above methods, compare with your "swinging answers" and see if they are comparable.

No matter which practice you settle on:
Double check your facts and re-test often.
Enjoy the practice, practice, practice.
Then what? Teach someone else.

#3. Standing on the Shoulders of Giants (Standing on Their Books) to Get a Better View.

We need a holistic approach to every animal, making sure that every facet of their lives is the best we can make it. Don't trust internet information 100%, please. Check out your own answers—easy as 1, 2, 3.

Out of all the books I have used for research—here are my top choices. These 10 authors have helped me save hundreds of lives. Without any doubt, when you add your resolve; we will be saving thousands more. In all these years as student, teacher, pioneer, first responder, and last house on the block before euthanasia; I know essential ingredients to success are: intention, purpose, and a few good books...

Bach, M.D., Edward and F. J. Wheeler, M.D. *The Bach Flower Remedies.* New Canaan: Keats Publishing Inc., 1979.

Boericke, M.D., William. *Materia Medica* Santa Rosa, CA: Boericke and Taffel, Inc. 1927.

Busch, Heather and Silver, Burton. *Why Cats Paint*. Berkley, CA: Ten Speed Press, 1994 (Has nothing to do with Essences, I just love the cats' paintings.)

Emoto, Masuru. *The Hidden Messages in Water*. Translated by David Thayne. New York: Atria Books, 2004.

Foster, Steven and Christopher Hobbs. *A Field Guide to Western Medicinal Plants and Herbs*. Boston: Houghton Mifflin Company, 2002.

Gerber, M.D., Richard. *A Practical Guide to Vibrational Medicine*. New York: Harper Collins Publishers, 2001. (Not any other version—as it was edited and sanitized in later editions.)

Kohanov, Linda. *The Tao of Equus*. Novato, CA: New World Library, 2001.

Keyes, Ken. *The Hundredth Monkey*. Vision Books, 1984

Palika, Liz. *The Complete Idiot's Guide to Natural Health for Dogs and Cats*. ALPHA, 2011.

Pryor, Karen. *Reaching The Animal Mind*. Scribner, 2010.

Wood, Matthew. *The Book of Herbal Wisdom: Using Plants as Medicines*. Berkeley: North Atlantic Books, 1997.

Wood, Matthew. *Vitalism: The History of Herbalism, Homeopathy, and Flower Essences*. Berkeley: North Atlantic Books, 2005.

On the Wrong Right Track

Don't be intimidated by anyone's credentials or sophistication or bank balance or public image or the magnitude of their industry. Here is one example of a David and a Goliath. I had been asked to participate in a research study at a prestigious zoo aimed at increasing activity of their Lions, Tigers, and Cheetahs for the entertainment of the public. I wanted the zoo to use my Flower Essences but they wanted to use my products containing medicinal-grade Lavender essential oil. The doctor told me these big Cats were physiologically the same as domestic Cats after I told him exposure to Lavender oil was a detriment to their health. He then told me they had poured Lavender oil on some plants—near the public viewing area—and the big Cats loved rolling in and sleeping in it. Here is my follow-up letter.

Dr. Zoo, (not his real name)   March 14, 2011

Thank you for the conversation on Friday. Sorry to be the bearer of the bad news concerning cats and oils but, with the onslaught of oils into the animal world touted as "natural and safe" hard evidence does exist of related illnesses and death. As I understand, cats do not have the enzymes (enzyme glucuronyl tranferases) necessary to eliminate build up of toxic metabolites caused by fragrances and certain oils like Tea Tree and Lavender. At the end is a short research article.

Additionally, essential oils are a severe drain on the planet's resources. Rose essential oil from Bulgaria (which I believe to be the best available in the world for uses in aromatherapy) requires 1,000 pounds of Rose petals to make 1 ounce of oil or 450 drops. Turkish Rose oil requires 250 pounds of petals for 1 ounce of oil. Either way, not economical or ecologically judicious while also considering the documented inhumane and deceitful practices in the perfume/fragrance industry.

Flower Essences and homeopathic Remedies I use:

- Require minimal amount of flowers, leaves, stems, etcetera, to make 1 gallon of Essence.
- Dosage is the same for a 14 pound Jack Russell dog as a 1,400 pound horse. Exact same = only several drops.
- Essences work 100% of the time—our success rate is 99% on all animals we attempt to help.
- Work permanently because Essences eliminate the root cause of the problem(s).
- No negative side effects.
- Proven successful helping in cases of abuse and animal cruelty as well as in rescuing during weeklong firestorms, and in the wide-reaching aftermath of the largest animal rescue in US history—caring for the victims of Hurricane Katrina.
- Proven on 15 species.
- Used on feral cats becoming friendly in less than 10 days. (One feral cat rescuer from Best Friends Sanctuary used ½ bottle of our Remedies created for Hurricane Katrina victims to trap, vet check, neuter, and adopt out 27 feral cats within one year = one ounce of Flower Essence Remedy.)

Problems such as shyness, aggression, marking, obsessive licking, and anxious behaviors are all remedied by the exact same formulas successfully used on the Katrina victims and thousands since 2005.

In my experience, shy and reticent behaviors are the result of either:

- Lingering, subtle depression or disappointment,
- Post-traumatic stress
- Insecurity, Anxiety, or
- Environmental dissatisfaction.

I rarely advise changing the environment since, as in the case of Katrina rescue efforts, it was impossible to alter the situation nonetheless, the animals did adjust, overcome fears, insecurities, accept their new surroundings, new schedules, food, and new caretakers. These same blends are used in shelters, sanctuaries, and hospital settings where situations are not optimum yet the animals overcome negative behaviors.

In households using Flower Essences, shy cats quit running away when company arrives, cats emerge from under beds or inside closets to explore the house as never before—even in broad daylight—even when there are people in the house! Even if the chronic behavior has been ongoing for years. As they feel less vulnerable and become more self-assured; they begin to explore and interact with family members and strangers alike. These changes are permanent and quick: 3-14 days unless in-bred or similarly damaged which could take 3-6 weeks.

I did begin researching a new formula for your Lions, Tigers, and Cheetahs but, want to make sure I have pinpointed your exact needs. One more conversation would be greatly appreciated.

My best,
Meg

FOLLOW-UP ON THE FOLLOW-UP—Never heard from him again after he asked for more "peer reviewed studies"—which I did supply to him. Good news is that all traces of this "study of oils to increase the zoo's big cats' activity during public visiting hours" was removed from their official website and never mentioned again.

ONE MORE FOLLOW-UP—What I am saying here is err on the side of caution when it comes to conflicting information. Many will argue for the benefits of oils for cats and to them, I say: re-read my letter to Dr. Zoo.

Against All Odds

Stand up for what is right and you will never be wrong.

Don't be afraid of terribly rich animal industries because many are terrible. Breeding for vanity and sport, manipulative breeding to meet a set standard, farming industry and slaughter house practices, veal Calves, Horses used for the pregnant mare urine. Then we have poor practices in ONLY SOME zoos, circuses, marine parks, rodeos, research animals, shelters, and the horrific ongoing plight of the American Mustang. Whether to fight terrorism, child abuse, violence, exploitation, or whatever you feel is not right, feel empowered that if you see something, say something.

On a local level, maybe it is the policies of the animal shelter where you volunteer that you find difficult. Many people have tried to introduce Flower Essences and other "new" ideas to the powers that be... be in control of decision making. Many have been met with negativity, what I think happens is that the people feel threatened that what they are doing now will be proven wrong. That's not it—ego and politics aside—if there is a better way; why not try? Do what many people do: spray themselves down first and then go inside to work.

Seemingly Hopeless is Far from Hopeless

The most difficult thought, emotion, feeling is hopelessness. Hopelessness is defined as having no expectation of good or success. Despair that takes your breath away making you sink to your knees. To give up and cave to the demands of isolation takes the life force from your blood. I have been there and I do not want to ever be there again. What I have been offered, during 40 years with Essences, is optimism. Anticipating the best of the best. Maybe with a slight limp or a patch of fur missing, but alive and well with a story to tell. Surround yourself with people that make a positive difference.

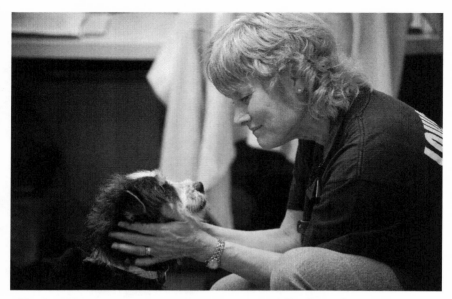

Charlene is one more person saving one more life. She is the quintessential
volunteer at any shelter, rescue, or sanctuary that needs her.

Indulge me one story here. The day we met was about 2 months
after Katrina struck Charlene's hometown of New Orleans where
abandoned animals were still being rescued. This day it was a fish. The
18" fish had been in a house for 8-10 weeks with no fresh water, food
or electricity to work the pump which essentially acted as this fish's
Iron Lung. The fish was in dire shape. His companions were dead and
he was almost there. We added fresh tap water, then worried about the
quality of the water, then added bottled water, then thought maybe he
was a salt water fish. With our help, he was fading faster than when he
was surviving on his own.

Charlene called the zoo and a vet answered, telling her to bring the
fish right over, the gates would be opened for her. She put the makeshift
tank in the backseat of her snazzy red convertible Mustang and drove
through the familiar streets like it was the emergency it was. The vets
said she saved the life of the fish. Not by her immediate response but in

driving so fast, she sloshed the water and the fish around so much that she re-energized both.

The fish lived. Charlene learned fish CPR and taught it to the rest of us. Yes, I'm serious. You take the fish gently around the body, glide it forward through the water, then pull gently backwards which forces the gills open. Repeat until the fish wants to wiggle away and resume 'breathing' on its own.

Thank you to all the Charlenes of the World… for every thing you do… every single day. Many animals have forever homes because of efforts like Charlene's and countless others.

Not Too Proud to Beg

Research monkeys, lab rats, and slaughterhouse animals FEEL MORE PAIN WATCHING others being tortured than when they are actually being tortured themselves. Let's hook up some of those same monitors to teenagers. Witnessing violence at home, in their neighborhoods, at school, on the internet, and in personal relationships negatively impacts our youth on a daily basis and with dire outcomes. Adults suffer too since many are stuck in their own personal teenage passageways never having fully reached emotional maturity with the ability or promise of making wise choices.

For better or worse, good or bad, behaviors change to adapt to the existing environment.

Teenagers are a national crisis and we all need to own up to that. Teenagers and damaged animals act out in similar fashions: aggressive, passive, or passive-aggressive. This comprehensive reaction to life molds their personalities and their expectations for all their days. Why does it happen? I have a theory. Lack of attention, praise, and role models shaping optimal behaviors.

How can this change?
1. Turn off the electronics for a few hours. Not asking for the impossible. Just a few hours.
2. Establish some guidelines or boundaries for the adolescents in your life. Not only your own but the ones you come in contact with during any given day. Look young people in the eye. Ask them to do something. Make them accountable for their actions—or inactions as the case may be.

3. Work increases the sense of belonging, sense of contribution, sense of positive self-worth and overall well-being. The consequences of not promoting the best traits in each young person often brings dire consequences, as played out every day in every city as suicide, bullying, victimization, and becoming invisible, those individuals disappearing right in front of our eyes. Threats and intimidation are a huge part of bullying, daily carrying over the insecurity and anxiety of being a target or a witness.

4. Use Flower Essences to hasten the recovery—a simple and immediate answer.

Worth the Risk.

If you suspected physical illness; you'd go to any length to help, then go there for mental and emotional health.

Take action:

1. Talk, plead, beg to find out the truth—THEIR TRUTH.
2. Privacy is a privilege. Snooping may be considered caring.
3. Children will seldom "rat out" people, for fear of retaliation. But true friends, caring adults, and brave Guardians will. Pick up the phone with your concerns. Walk into a room looking for answers. Ask questions. Don't take "Nothing's wrong" and "I dunno" as answers.
4. Find successfully proven therapists and programs. One high school student as a black-out drinker skated past a licensed psychiatrist, 2 school counselors, 6 teachers, coaches, other parents, and a court appointed drug and alcohol counselor.

What do you have to lose?

Horrifying statistics surround adolescent suicide, homicide, addiction, self-mutilation, abuse, at-risk activities, and personality disorders. Here is just one statistic: 15% of 10-19 year old children have thought IN DETAIL how to kill themselves. Right now, imagine

100 children, and ask: who are the "15" FIFTEEN with thoughts IN DETAIL on how to kill themselves? You can make a difference, never doubt that.

Rites of Passage Remedy

Here is an extensive Flower Essence blend for helping bullies, victims including bystanders (remember the pain felt by animals witnessing cruelty) and shunning where victims are ignored in public and/or left out of social activities including the large-scale impact of social media. These Essences were carefully chosen to treat the cause with its need to aggressively or passively act out, as well as its effects upon everyone involved including family and friends—victims and witnesses alike. Anyone can use this remedy while actively pursuing activities to increase positive self-esteem. Watch the change as new patterns of learning and behaving are established, bringing out the best qualities in each person.

Aconite (overcome sensitivity and restlessness), Agrimony (draw out the authentic personality), Angel's Trumpet (acquire confident outlook), Apple (cleanses negative self-image), Clematis (for focus and follow-through), Impatiens (for patience, composure, and tolerance), Mustard (reduce lingering depression), Rose (create positive self-sufficiency), Sweetgrass (open up dialogue and welcome change), and Yarrow (thrive in a negative environment).

If you have a young person or someone you love behind locked doors either actual or figuratively—use this blend yourself as well and start a new dialogue. Only you can imagine what you have to lose. If you suspect there is a problem; bet your last dollar that there is one.

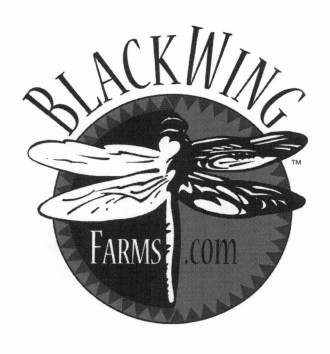

BlackWingFarms.com
760-728-9900

34875477R00104

Made in the USA
Lexington, KY
22 August 2014